POL KOENIG'S
BASIC BOOK OF VITAMIN HEALTH

If you would like to receive our current
catalogue and announcements of new titles, please
send your name and address to:

ROBERT DAVIES PUBLISHING,
P.O. Box 702, Outremont, Quebec,
Canada H2V 4N6

POL KOENIG'S
BASIC BOOK OF VITAMIN HEALTH

BY POL KOENIG, WITH NICOLE MARCHAL
TRANSLATED BY MADELEINE HÉBERT

ROBERT DAVIES PUBLISHING
MONTREAL/TORONTO

TABLE OF CONTENTS

PART ONE:
VITAMINS   **9**

PART TWO:
MINERALS AND TRACE ELEMENTS   **113**

TABLES

PART ONE: VITAMINS

INTRODUCTION

The human body cannot synthesize vitamins, and so they must be included in our daily food intake. This poses no problem if our daily diets are nutritionally balanced. Unfortunately, although we talk a lot about nutrition, we do not think about *malnutrition* in the modern Western world, and yet this remains a problem. In fact, many daily diets are not well balanced, because much of the food processed in modern factories has lost so many essential nutrients. For instance, if we could replace the great quantities of white sugar that we consume with honey or non-refined brown sugar, we would not need to take fluoride supplements to help prevent tooth decay. There is also a general preference in our society for white bread, even though whole-wheat bread contains much more fibre, wheat germ, and essential vitamins.

All this raises many questions about vitamins, and the important role they play in our lives.

1.

QUESTIONS ABOUT VITAMINS

1.
WHAT ARE VITAMINS?

The word vitamin comes from *vita* (life) and *amino* (organic molecule.) Vitamins are defined as organic molecules that are found in very small amounts (except vitamin F) in a well-balanced diet, that have no energy value, but that are essential for life.

2
WHEN WERE VITAMINS FIRST DISCOVERED?

The term vitamin was coined in 1910, following observation of certain pathological conditions, such as beriberi[1] and scurvy[2].

3.
WHAT ROLE DO VITAMINS PLAY?

Vitamins are necessary for the development and maintenance of healthy bodies and organs. They participate in a series of biochemical reactions that occur in the body, and often act in synergy with minerals and trace elements.

4.
HOW MANY VITAMINS ARE THERE?

It is difficult to know exactly how many vitamins there are, because new ones are being discovered as science progresses. Vitamins are usually identified by letters of the alphabet, and the principal ones we know of are vitamin A, vitamins of the B-complex group, vitamin C, vitamin D, vitamin E, vitamin F, vitamin K, and vitamin P.

5.
HOW ARE VITAMINS CLASSIFIED?

Vitamins are divided into two general categories, according to their properties:

1- *Fat-soluble vitamins, which can be stored by the body*

2- *Water-soluble vitamins, which are not stored by the body*

This is an important distinction. Vitamins A and D, for example, can be stored for a few weeks, but the body must receive new supplies of vitamins such as B, C, and P frequently.

Fat-soluble vitamins stored by the body:		Water-soluble vitamins not stored by the body:
A, D, E, F, K		B-complex, C, P

6.
WHEN SHOULD WE CONSIDER VITAMIN THERAPY?

Therapeutic vitamin supplements could be recommended to *almost everyone* twice a year–in the spring and in the fall. This is because seasonal changes have a tendency to upset internal energy balance.

However, if the questionnaire in chapter 2 reveals certain vitamin deficiencies, these should be treated separately, regardless of the season. In any case, daily minimum intake levels of vitamins and mineral supplements should always be maintained.

7.
HOW LONG DOES VITAMIN THERAPY LAST?

A one-month treatment is generally advised, but this should be adapted for individual cases, and should take into consideration specific physiological conditions (pregnancy, menopause, adolescence, etc.).

8.
WHICH VITAMINS ARE RECOMMENDED?

You can find out if you have any vitamin deficiencies by answering the questions in chapter 2. However, daily dosages of vitamins B, C, and P are advisable for everyone, as these are not retained by the body.

9.

DOES TODAY'S LIFESTYLE
AFFECT VITAMINS?

Various features of modern life can have a disturbing effect on some people. An unreasonable or unbalanced diet, use of tobacco or alcohol, excessive stress, or disruption of the natural cycles of rest, work, and recreation can cause "pathological fatigue."

Some examples:

9A.

When sugar is refined, it loses some of its vitamins, notably A, B_2, B_3, B_5, B_6, D, and E.

9B.

Refined flour and white bread contain ten times fewer vitamins and minerals than the whole-wheat varieties.

9C.

Certain food additives and colorings can have serious side effects, destroying vitamins B_6, B_1, D. and E.

9D.

Alcohol, coffee, tobacco, and oral contraceptives often cause vitamin depletion:
- Alcohol: vitamin A and B-complex vitamins
- Coffee: vitamin A and B-complex vitamins
- Tobacco: B-complex vitamins and vitamin C
- Oral contraceptives: B-complex vitamins, vitamin C, and vitamin E

9E.

Some medications have a negative affect on vitamins:
- Laxatives, diuretics, and mineral oil (paraffin) destroy vitamins B_{12}, D, E, and K
- Antibiotics destroy vitamins C, K, and P

- Cortisone destroys vitamins C and P
- Aspirin destroys vitamins C, K, and P
- Sleeping pills destroy B-complex vitamins and vitamin D

9F.

X-rays destroy vitamins F and K.

Avoiding the above-mentioned items is the best way to prevent vitamin loss. However, when this is not possible, augmenting dosages of specific vitamins can help to compensate for their loss.

10.

WHO REQUIRES ADDITIONAL VITAMINS?

- Good nutrition is of primary importance if you are either pregnant or breast-feeding
- Anyone to whom the lists in section 9 (above) apply. For example, smokers need 30% more vitamin C. Even then, they remain more vulnerable to flu infections
- Teen-agers require more vitamin A for growth and vitamin D for bone calcium
- Athletically active people need more of certain vitamins, depending on which sports they practise

- Older people need vitamins F, E, D, and B-complex vitamins, in this order of importance
- Patients recovering from surgery
- People who are under stress
- People on a weight-loss diet

11.

WHAT CAN I DO?

General nutritional awareness is better than it was ten or twenty years ago. Vitamin-rich, wholesome foods such as whole-wheat bread, hearty soups, and fresh fruits and vegetables are back in fashion. In addition, many people today either avoid alcohol completely or have reduced their alcohol consumption.

Turning to health foods is a positive reaction against artificial products and chemical additives. While the apples from our backyard trees may be uneven in shape or colour, they are much better for us than the 'perfect' apples found in the supermarket. Commercial produce may look attractive, but often it has been heavily treated and is of poorer nutritional quality.

In this book, you will find details about dietary supplements that can help to correct nutritional and vitamin deficiencies. Keep in mind that this information is offered for your consideration and reflection, and is not intended to replace your physician's advice. However, we hope this guide will enable you to make more informed choices regarding nutrition, and will help you along the path to better health.

Notes

1. Scurvy is a disease that was common among sailors who ate only canned foods. It was discovered that scurvy is caused by a lack of vitamin C.

2. Beriberi is a disease common to people who eat only polished (white) rice. It was discovered that beriberi is caused by a lack of vitamin B_{12}.

2

THE EASY-CHEK® VITAMIN-DEFICIENCY TEST

ANSWER THE TEST QUESTIONS BY
INDICATING TO THE RIGHT OF
EACH QUESTION THE NUMBER
THAT BEST DESCRIBES
YOUR CIRCUMSTANCES:

0 = NO OR NEVER

1 = SOMETIMES

2 = YES OR OFTEN

VITAMIN A

1. Do you have painful menstrual cramps? _____
2. Do you have problems seeing in the dark? _____
3. Are your eyes tired or irritated? _____
4. Do you have dry or rough skin? _____
5. Is your tooth enamel weak? _____

Vitamin A - subtotal _____

VITAMIN B

6. Do you experience pins and needles in your legs? _____
7. Are you tired or anxious? _____
8. Do you suffer from constipation? _____
9. Have you experienced memory loss? _____
10. Are you losing your hair? _____

Vitamin B-complex - subtotal _____

VITAMIN C

11. If you cut yourself, does the wound heal easily?_____
12. Do you often have a cold or a sore throat?_____
13. Do you smoke more than 10 cigarettes a day?_____
14. Is your complexion very pallid? _____
15. Do you have allergies? _____

Vitamin C - subtotal _____

VITAMIN D

16. Do your nails break easily?_____
17. Are you shortsighted? _____
18. Do you have insomnia?_____
19. Are you prone to diarrhea?_____
20. Have you ever broken any bones?_____

Vitamin D - subtotal _____

VITAMIN E

21. Do you have sore or tired muscles?_____
22. Have you experienced any hair loss? _____
23. Do you have high cholesterol? _____
24. Do you have migraines or headaches? _____
25. Do you take oral contraceptives, or have vaginal or genital problems? _____

Vitamin E - subtotal _____

VITAMIN F

26. Do you have dry skin or acne?_____
27. Have you ever had a heart attack? _____
28. Do you have varicose veins or hemorrhoids? _____
29. Do you use normal cooking and salad oils?_____
30. Do you take medication at least once a week?_____

Vitamin F - subtotal _____

WRITE YOUR TOTAL HERE

A.
INTERPRETING YOUR RESULTS

Once you have answered all the questions, add up the results to obtain your subtotals by vitamin and your grand total. If your grand total is:

• **Less than 15**: You are in good shape, but remain vigilant about your diet and your health.

• **15 through 35**: It is time to consider correcting nutritional imbalances.

• **Over 35**: You should consult your physician or a dietitian as soon as possible.

Regardless of your results, refer to section B following the table.

DISTRIBUTION OF VITAMIN SCORES

	Vit. A	Vit. B	Vit. C	Vit. D	Vit. E	Vit. F
	10	10	10	10	10	10
	7	7	7	7	7	7
	5	5	5	5	5	5
	3	3	3	3	3	3
	0	0	0	0	0	0

B.
COMPLETING YOUR TEST ANALYSIS

Transcribe your test **subtotals** to the appropriate columns in the preceding table. This will enable you to analyze each vitamin category, and to supplement your diet accordingly.

• **If your subtotals are 1 to 3 in all categories**: You are in good health, although evaluating your diet could still be beneficial.

• **If your subtotal is 4 to 7 in any category**: You should correct specific deficiencies with a few dietary supplements.

• **If your subtotal is 8 to 10**: You have severe deficiencies, and should seek medical attention.

Please read carefully the following summary before proceeding:

DEFICIENCIES AND REMEDIES

Deficiency of:	Can be corrected by taking:
Vitamin A	Carrot capsules
VItamin B	Brewer's yeast
Vitamin C	Acerola or rose-hip capsules
Vitamin D	Halibut-liver oil
Vitamin E	Wheat germ or natural vitamin E capsules
Vitamin F	Borage or evening-primrose capsules

3.

VITAMINS AND THEIR PROPERTIES

VITAMIN A

Retinol or provitamin A (beta-carotene)
Growth vitamin
Fat-soluble

1. FUNCTIONS

• Essential for good vision, particularly night vision
• Keeps skin and mucous membranes healthy
• Aids growth
• Facilitates assimilation of fats (lipids)
• Acts as a defense against germs and provides better resistance to infection
• Helps counter toxic agents in the environment
• Scientific studies show a possible connection between vitamin A deficiency and certain types of cancer

2. RECOMMENDED DAILY ALLOWANCE

0.5 to 1.8 mg (1,500 to 5,400 IU[1])

3. SOURCES

Provitamin A in fruit and vegetables:

• 1 raw carrot (10,000 IU)

VITAMIN A

- 100 grams of melon (3,400 IU)[1]
- 1 cup of dried apricots (16,000 IU)
- 100 grams of dandelion greens (14,000 IU)
- 100 grams of blueberries (1.6 mg)

Vitamin A in animal products:

- 100 grams of calf liver (30,000 IU)
- 100 grams of cod- or halibut-liver oil (from 85,000 IU to 2.40 million IU)
- Dairy products: butter, milk, and cheese

4. EFFECTS OF VITAMIN A DEFICIENCY

- Allergies
- Pallid complexion
- Loss of appetite
- Dull, dry hair
- Irritated eyes
- Diminished sense of smell
- Night blindness and vision problems
- Dry, rough skin
- Sinus problems
- Weak tooth enamel
- Diminished resistance to infection
- Painful menstruation
- Cancer (respiratory tract, bladder, stomach, prostate, etc.)

5. DESTROYED OR INHIBITED BY

- Alcohol
- Coffee
- Cortisone
- Light
- Oxygen
- Vitamin D deficiency
- Excess iron and copper (from cooking utensils)

6. SPECIFIC APPLICATIONS

- Vision problems
- Acne
- Alcoholism
- Allergies
- Arthritis
- Regular athletic activity
- Sinusitis
- Stress
- Living or working in a polluted environment
- Dental problems
- Cystitis
- Diabetes
- Eczema
- Cardiac condition
- Hepatitis
- Headaches
- Psoriasis

7. NATURAL DIETARY SUPPLEMENTS

- Provitamin A, or carrot oil in capsules or flakes
- Halibut-liver-oil capsules (containing B-complex and D vitamins)
- Pollen granules
- Alfalfa sprouts

8. RECOMMENDATIONS

- Vision disorders can be reduced through occasional therapy with carrot-oil capsules.

- To prepare your skin for tanning and to keep your tan after vacation, take carrot-oil capsules.

- Treatment with halibut-liver oil is effective because its combination of vitamins A and D helps prevent hypervitaminosis. It is important to be aware that an accumulation of vitamin A in the body can cause critical hypervitaminosis.

- Excess accumulation of fat-soluble vitamin A is dangerous and could lead to appetite loss or even cirrhosis. It is always best to be safe; consult your physician or dietitian for advice about therapeutic supplements.

- Do not prepare raw vegetables more than two hours in advance. Light and air are the enemies of vitamin A.

• People who must sit for long hours in front of cathode-ray screens (televisions, computer monitors) should increase their vitamin A intake.

Note

1. IUs are international units, used to express the biological activity of vitamins. They are an alternative to expression by unit of mass (micrograms, milligrams, etc.).

VITAMIN B₁

Also known as thiamine or aneurin
Nervous-system vitamin
Water-soluble

1. FUNCTIONS

• Controls the metabolism of glucose (sugars), lipids (fats), and amino acids (major factors in protein development)
• Helps to control neural transmission, reduces stress

2. RECOMMENDED DAILY ALLOWANCE

1 to 2 mg

3. SOURCES

• Whole-grain cereals
• Brazil nuts (1 cup = 3 mg)
• Brewer's yeast (2 tbsp = 3 mg)
• Egg yolks
• Milk

4. EFFECTS OF VITAMIN B₁ DEFICIENCY

- Depression
- Digestive disorders
- Circulatory, visual or mental problems
- Beriberi (see chapter 1, section 2)

5. DESTROYED OR INHIBITED BY

- Alcohol
- Sulfates
- Stress
- Surgery
- Antibiotics
- Excess sugar

6. SPECIFIC APPLICATIONS

- Alcoholism
- Anemia
- Weak heart
- Diarrhea
- Diabetes
- Indigestion
- Stress
- Tachycardia

VITAMIN B1

VITAMIN B1

7. NATURAL DIETARY SUPPLEMENTS

- Brewer's yeast: 2 tbsp daily daily provides 3 mg of vitamin B1 (see chapter 4)
- Preservative-free natural cereals
- Wheat germ and wheat-germ oil (see chapter 4)

8. RECOMMENDATIONS

- Vitamin B1 is destroyed by the sulfates added to pre-cooked potatoes, instant mashed potatoes, shrimp, mustard, ice cream, white sugar, and beer.
- Pregnant women require 4.5 mg of vitamin B1 daily.
- People who often eat sweets should increase their vitamin B1 intake.

VITAMIN B2

Also known as riboflavi n or lactoflavin
Provides energy, prevents muscle cramps
Water-soluble

1. FUNCTIONS

• Active in the formation of enzymes in respiration
• Regulates digestion, iron fixing in the blood, hormonal metabolism (stimulates insulin production)
• Improves vision

2. RECOMMEND ED D AILY ALLOWANCE

1.5 to 2.5 mg

3. SOURCES

• Milk
• Brewer' yeast (3 tbsp = 1 mg)
• Eggs
• Cheese
• Almonds (1 cup = 1 mg)
• Beef liver

VITAMIN B2

4. EFFECTS OF VITAMIN B$_2$ DEFICIENCY

- Cataracts
- Dizziness
- Vertigo
- Eye infections
- Growth retardation
- Tongue chancres

5. DESTROYED OR INHIBITED BY

- Oral contraceptives
- Antibiotics
- Too much glucose (sugar)
- Tobacco
- Alcohol

6. SPECIFIC APPLICATIONS

- Vertigo
- Chronic digestive disorders
- Dermatosis
- Oral inflammation
- Photophobia (hypersensitivity to light)
- Growth disorders
- Acne
- Alcoholism
- Arthritis

- Cataracts
- Stress
- Diabetes
- Diarrhea

7. NATURAL DIETARY SUPPLEMENTS

- Brewer's yeast (see chapter 4)
- Beef-liver capsules
- Preservative-free whole-wheat bread with yeast

8. RECOMMENDATIONS

- Including bean sprouts in your regular diet is a good health habit.
- People with a vitamin B2 deficiency should limit their intake of millet.

VITAMIN B2

VITAMIN B3

Also known as niacin (nicotinic acid)
Increases energy
Water-soluble

1. FUNCTIONS

• Vital for the digestive system, healthy skin, and good circulation
• Reduces stress and cholesterol levels

2. RECOMMENDED DAILY ALLOWANCE

10 to 20 mg

3. SOURCES

• Brewer's yeast
• Tofu
• Calf liver
• Lean meats
• Fish
• Cereals
• Soybeans

4. EFFECTS OF VITAMIN B3 DEFICIENCY

- Appetite loss
- Depression
- Fatigue
- Headaches
- Insomnia
- Nausea
- Skin problems
- Nervous disorders

5. DESTROYED OR INHIBITED BY

- Meat
- Coffee
- Alcohol
- Antibiotics

6. SPECIFIC APPLICATIONS

- Fatigue
- Insomnia
- Memory loss
- Nervousness
- Anxiety
- Appetite loss
- Dermatosis
- Sore muscles

VITAMIN B3

VITAMIN B3

- Gastrointestinal disorders
- Sun sensitivity

7. NATURAL DIETARY SUPPLEMENTS

- Brewer's yeast (see Chapter 4)
- Whole-wheat bread with yeast
- Wheat germ, wheat-germ oil

8. RECOMMENDATION

- People who are allergic to the sun (hypersensitive skin) should consider a two-month therapeutic treatment of vitamin B3 before exposing themselves to UV rays. After treatment, begin with short periods of sun exposure, lengthening the time gradually and within reason.

VITAMIN B5

Also known as pantothenic acid
For skin and hair
Water-soluble

1. FUNCTIONS

- Essential for childhood and teenage growth, the formation of cells, adrenalin production, healing wounds, and the development of antibodies to fight infection
- Required by the central nervous system
- Reduces side effects of antibiotics

2. RECOMMENDED DAILY ALLOWANCE

6 to 10 mg

3. SOURCES

- Avocados
- Salmon
- Royal jelly
- Brewer's yeast (9.5 mg per 100 g)
- Cooked mushrooms
- Lamb

VITAMIN B5

4. EFFECTS OF VITAMIN B5 DEFICIENCY

- Diarrhea
- Eczema
- Hypoglycemia
- Hair loss
- Muscle cramps
- Premature aging
- Vomiting
- Fatigue

5. DESTROYED OR INHIBITED BY

- Alcohol
- Coffee
- Aspirin
- Stress
- Antibiotics

6. SPECIFIC APPLICATIONS

- Fatigue
- Weak muscles
- Low resistance to infection
- Vomiting
- Diarrhea

- Low blood pressure
- Hypoglycemia
- Hair loss
- Eczema
- Stomach aches

7. NATURAL DIETARY SUPPLEMENTS

- Royal jelly (see chapter 4)
- Brewer's yeast (see chapter 4)
- Pollen (see chapter 4)
- Wheat germ (see chapter 4)

8. RECOMMENDATION

- For hair loss, treatment should consist of vitamin B_5, taken in conjunction with vitamin B_{17} (biotin) or vitamin H.

VITAMIN B6

Also known as pyridoxine (sometimes known as vitamin G)
Required by meat eaters
Water-soluble

1. FUNCTIONS

- Helps regulate protein metabolism
- Stabilizes iron in the blood

2. RECOMMENDED DAILY ALLOWANCE

2 mg to 150 mg

3. SOURCES

- Liver
- Avocados
- Bananas
- Wheat germ
- Brewer's yeast
- Brown rice (1 cup = 2 mg)

4. EFFECTS OF VITAMIN B6 DEFICIENCY

- Acne
- Anemia
- Arthritis
- Depression
- Hair loss
- Inability to concentrate
- Vertigo

5. DESTROYED OR INHIBITED BY

- Alcohol
- Oral contraceptives
- Tobacco
- Coffee
- X-rays

6. SPECIFIC APPLICATIONS

- Menstrual cramps
- Hair loss
- Fatigue
- Listlessness
- Depression
- Nervousness
- Conjunctivitis
- Acne

VITAMIN B6

- Memory loss
- Poor assimilation of vitamin B_{12}
- Cystitis
- Hypoglycemia
- Sun sensitivity

7. NATURAL DIETARY SUPPLEMENTS

- Brewer's yeast (see Chapter 4)
- Wheat germ

8. RECOMMENDATIONS

- Vitamin B_6 requirements increase according to the amount of animal protein contained in the diet.
- Vitamin B_6 should be taken to counter the effects of exposure to X-rays.
- Vitamin B_6 helps relieve premenstrual tension and problems associated with menopause.

VITAMIN B7

Inositol (also known as vitamin I or vitamin J)
Water-soluble

1. FUNCTIONS

- Controls cholesterol levels
- Helps maintain healthy hair, prevents hair loss

2. RECOMMENDED DAILY ALLOWANCE

100 mg

3. SOURCES

- Wheat germ
- Brewer's yeast
- Soya
- Whole grain cereals
- Roasted peanuts with skin (1 cup = 400 mg)

4. EFFECTS OF VITAMIN B7 DEFICIENCY
- Elevated cholesterol levels
- Eczema
- Eye problems
- Hair loss

VITAMIN B7

5. DESTROYED OR INHIBITED BY

- Alcohol
- Coffee
- Antibiotics

6. SPECIFIC APPLICATIONS

- Hair loss
- Constipation
- Eczema
- High cholesterol
- Cardiac disease
- Obesity

7. NATURAL DIETARY SUPPLEMENTS

- Brewer's yeast (see chapter 4)
- Wheat germ (see chapter 4)
- Pollen (see chapter 4)

8. RECOMMENDATION

- Regular intake of brewer's yeast helps avoid short-term and long-term hair loss.

VITAMIN B9

Folic acid
Helps protect against anemia
Water-soluble

1. FUNCTIONS

- Has analgesic properties
- Aids protein metabolism and formation of red blood cells
- Plays a role in growth and reproduction

2. RECOMMENDED DAILY ALLOWANCE

0.01 to 0.4 mg

3. SOURCES

- Brewer's yeast (1 tbsp = 200 mg)
- Salad greens
- Dried dates
- Tuna fish
- Oysters
- Salmon
- Soya flour (430 mg per 100 g)

VITAMIN B9

4. EFFECTS OF VITAMIN B9 DEFICIENCY

- Anemia
- Digestive disorders
- Growth disorders
- Graying hair

5. DESTROYED OR INHIBITED BY

- Alcohol
- Coffee
- Tobacco
- Stress
- Antibiotics
- Sulfa drugs

6. SPECIFIC APPLICATIONS

- Appetite loss
- Gastro-intestinal disorders
- Alcoholism
- Fatigue
- Mental illness
- Stress
- Stomach ulcers
- Frequent hemorrhaging
- Chronic diarrhea

7. NATURAL DIETARY SUPPLEMENTS

- Wheat germ (see chapter 4)
- Brewer's yeast

8. RECOMMENDATIONS

- Vitamin B9 is recommended to help heal bone fractures.
- Pregnant women have an increased need for vitamin B9; in conjunction with iron, it helps prevent anemia.
- Vitamin B9 protects the body against toxins.

VITAMIN B10

Also known as para-aminobenzoic acid (PABA)
Anti-scelorodermic vitamin
Water-soluble

1. FUNCTIONS

- Facilitates assimilation of vitamin B5
- Regulates protein metabolism
- Assists in formation of blood cells

2. RECOMMENDED DAILY ALLOWANCE

10 to 100 mg

3. SOURCES

- Brewer's yeast (10 mg to 100 g)
- Natural whole grain cereals
- Liver
- Buttermilk (whey)
- Molasses and complete cane sugar
- Eggs
- Soybeans

4. EFFECTS OF VITAMIN B10 DEFICIENCY

- Constipation
- Depression
- Fatigue
- Gray hair
- Headaches
- Irritability

5. DESTROYED OR INHIBITED BY

- Alcohol
- Coffee
- Sulpha drugs

6. SPECIFIC APPLICATIONS

- Wrinkles
- Graying hair
- Sensitivity to UV rays
- Hyperthyroidism
- Sterility
- Stress
- Sunburn

VITAMIN B10

7. NATURAL DIETARY SUPPLEMENTS

- Brewer's yeast (see Chapter 4)
- Bean sprouts

8. RECOMMENDATIONS

- Vitamin B_{10} helps produce melanin, which protects the skin against the sun's harmful effects.

VITAMIN B12

Also known as cyanocobalamin
Helps in the formation of red blood cells
Water-soluble

1. FUNCTIONS

• Facilitates tissue regeneration and the metabolism
of fats, sugars, and proteins
• Essential for the formation of red blood cells

2. RECOMMENDED DAILY ALLOWANCE

3 mcg

3. SOURCES

• Beef liver
• Tuna fish
• Beef
• Eggs
• Corn
• Spirulina

VITAMIN B12

4. EFFECTS OF VITAMIN B$_{12}$ DEFICIENCY

- General weakness
- Nervousness
- Movement and speech difficulties
- Mental illness

5. DESTROYED OR INHIBITED BY

- Vegetarian diet
- Vitamin B$_6$ deficiency
- Alcohol
- Coffee
- Tobacco
- Laxatives
- Oral contraceptives

6. SPECIFIC APPLICATIONS

- Fatigue
- General weakness
- Nervousness
- Appetite loss
- Speech disorders
- Diarrhea
- Mood swings
- Alcoholism

7. NATURAL DIETARY SUPPLEMENTS

- Spirulina
- Tamari (Japanese soy sauce)
- Shoyu (soy sauce fermented with wheat)

8. RECOMMENDATION

• Since lactic fermentation helps the body synthesize vitamin B_{12}, strict vegetarians who avoid dairy products should take this vitamin to remedy deficiencies.

VITAMIN B12

VITAMIN B15

Also known as panganic acid
Vitamin for athletes
Water-soluble

1. FUNCTIONS

• Plays an essential role in cellular respiration, and in the metabolic processes of the muscles, kidneys, and liver
  • Lowers cholesterol
  • Protects the liver against cirrhosis
  • Fights fatigue and retards cellular aging
  • Improves athletic performance

2. RECOMMENDED DAILY ALLOWANCE

50 to 150 mg

3. SOURCES

  • Brewer's yeast (128 mg per 100 g)
  • Brown rice and corn
  • Sunflower and sesame seeds

4. EFFECTS OF VITAMIN B₁₅ DEFICIENCY

- Cardiovascular diseases
- Fatigue
- Glandular and nervous disorders

5. DESTROYED OR INHIBITED BY

- Alcohol
- Coffee
- Heat from cooking

6. SPECIFIC APPLICATIONS

- Alcoholism
- Asthma
- High cholesterol
- Insomnia
- Fatigue
- Rheumatism
- Athletic endurance

7. NATURAL DIETARY SUPPLEMENTS

- Brewer's yeast (see chapter 4)
- Wheat germ

VITAMIN B15

8. RECOMMENDATIONS

- Vitamin B15 has been widely studied in United States and Russia, and has proved to be beneficial for treating alcoholism and retardation.

VITAMIN B15

VITAMIN B$_{17}$

Also known as biotin (or vitamin H)
Hair and skin vitamin
Water-soluble

1. FUNCTIONS

• Regulates the synthesis of fatty acids, amino acids, and hemoglobin
• Facilitates absorption of other B vitamins

2. RECOMMENDED DAILY ALLOWANCE

0.3 mg

3. SOURCES

• Egg yolks (1 = 10 mcg)
• Brown rice
• Brewer's yeast (1 tablespoon = 20 mcg)
• Whole-grain cereals

4. EFFECTS OF VITAMIN B$_{17}$ DEFICIENCY

• Depression
• Dry skin

VITAMIN B17

- Fatigue
- Insomnia
- Muscular pain
- Appetite loss

5. DESTROYED OR INHIBITED BY

- Antibiotics
- Egg whites
- Alcohol
- Coffee
- Sulfa drugs

6. SPECIFIC APPLICATIONS

- Fatigue and sore muscles
- Appetite loss
- High cholesterol
- Depression
- Irritability

7. NATURAL DIETARY SUPPLEMENT

- Brewer's yeast (see chapter 4)

8. RECOMMENDATION
- Vitamin B17 is recommended for depression and for hair loss.

CHOLINE

Liver vitamin
Water-soluble

1. FUNCTIONS

- Lecithin formation
- Ensures neural transmission
- Metabolism of fats and cholesterol
- Regulates liver function

2. RECOMMENDED DAILY ALLOWANCE

100 mg

3. SOURCES

- Soybeans
- Egg yolks
- Lecithin
- Brewer's yeast
- Fish

CHOLINE

4. EFFECTS OF CHOLINE DEFICIENCY

- Stomach ulcers
- Growth disorders
- Hypertension
- Cardiovascular disorders

5. DESTROYED OR INHIBITED BY

- Heat from cooking
- Alcohol
- Coffee

6. SPECIFIC APPLICATIONS

- Alcoholism
- Baldness
- High cholesterol
- Constipation
- Headaches
- Insomnia
- Cardiovascular disorders
- Hypertension
- Hypoglycemia

7. NATURAL DIETARY SUPPLEMENT

- Brewer's yeast (see chapter 4)

8. RECOMMENDATION

- A diet rich in brewer's yeast or lecithin is recommended for liver problems and high cholesterol.

CHOLINE

VITAMIN C

Ascorbic acid
Water-soluble

1. FUNCTIONS

- Formation of teeth and bones
- Collagen production
- Helps heal burns and wounds
- Prevents hemorrhaging
- Increases resistance to infection
- Vitamin protection
- Anti-toxin
- Anti-anemic (encourages intestinal absorption of iron)
- Stimulates intellectual faculties
- Regulates metabolic and hormonal functions
- Increases male fertility
- Improves disposition
- Improves athletic performance

2. RECOMMENDED DAILY ALLOWANCE

60—120 mg to 5 g

3. SOURCES

- Fruit (oranges: 50 mg per 100 g; lemons: 45 mg per 100 g; black currants: 135 mg per 100 g)
- Green pepper, parsley (170 mg per 100 g)
- Vegetables (turnips, cabbage: 100 mg per 100 g)

4. EFFECTS OF VITAMIN C DEFICIENCY

- Anemia
- Bleeding gums
- Broken capillaries
- Slow healing
- Bruises
- Digestive problems
- Nose bleeds
- Allergies

5. DESTROYED OR INHIBITED BY

- Antibiotics
- Aspirin
- Cortisone
- Stress
- Tobacco
- High fever
- Light

VITAMIN C

VITAMIN C

- Heat (vitamin C is destroyed at temperatures exceeding 65°C)

6. SPECIFIC APPLICATIONS

- Alcoholism
- Allergies
- Arteriosclerosis
- Arthritis
- Baldness
- High cholesterol
- Colds
- Cystitis
- Hypoglycemia
- Cardiac ailments
- Hepatitis
- Insect bites
- Obesity
- Sinusitis
- Stress
- Dental cavities
- Back pain

7. NATURAL DIETARY SUPPLEMENTS

- Acerola or rose hips (25% vitamin C)
- Phytotherapy is very helpful to increase vitamin C–hibiscus, black currant, horseradish, evening primrose (cynorhodon), dandelion, sallow-thorn. Vegeta-

bles such as garlic, parsley, and watercress also offer appreciable quantities of vitamin C.

8. RECOMMENDATIONS

• Since vitamin C is water-soluble, it can be wasted when cooking water is discarded. Soups are healthy because they retain their vitamin content.

• People who suffer from insomnia should only take vitamin C in its natural form.

• Smokers require 30% more vitamin C than non-smokers.

• Vitamin C must be taken every day. It is important to remember that it can be assimilated two hours after a meal.

• Humans are one of the few animals whose regular diet must include vitamin C, as they are incapable of producing it naturally.

• Women who take oral contraceptives should increase their vitamin C intake.

VITAMIN C

VITAMIN D

Also known as cholecalciferol
Prevents rickets
Fat-soluble

1. FUNCTIONS

• Regulates calcium and phosphorus metabolism (bone formation)
• Reduces stress
• Increases immunity
• Protects the heart
• Maintains normal proportion of blood coagulants
• Beneficial for the skin

2. RECOMMENDED DAILY ALLOWANCE

0.01 mg (400 to 1,500 IU)

3. SOURCES

• Sunlight (UV rays react with a substance present in the skin)
• Fish oils (10,000 IU per 100 g)
• Egg yolks (265 IU per 100 g)
• Sardines in oil (1,380 IU per 100 g)

- Mushrooms
- Milk

4. EFFECTS OF VITAMIN D DEFICIENCY

- Burning sensations in the throat and mouth
- Diarrhea
- Insomnia
- Myopia
- Nervousness
- Problems with teeth and bones (rickets, etc.)
- Brittle nails

5. DESTROYED OR INHIBITED BY

- Sleeping pills and barbiturates
- Laxatives and diuretics
- Certain mineral oils
- Air pollution

6. SPECIFIC APPLICATIONS

- Acne
- Alcoholism
- Allergies
- Arthritis
- Cystitis
- Eczema

VITAMIN D

- Psoriasis
- Stress

7. NATURAL DIETARY SUPPLEMENTS

- Halibut-liver oil is 50 times richer in vitamins A and D than is cod-liver oil

8. RECOMMENDATIONS

- Vitamin D therapy is recommended for people who are not exposed to natural sunlight, for night guards, and for inhabitants of polluted areas where smog filters out UV rays.
- Since vitamin D deficiency is often noted in newborns, increased intake is recommended during pregnancy.

VITAMIN E

Also known as tocopherol
Fat-soluble

1. FUNCTIONS

- Retards aging through anti-oxidizing action
- Anticoagulant
- Lowers blood cholesterol
- Fortifies capillaries
- Protects lungs against pollution
- Repairs muscles and nerves
- Increases fertility

2. RECOMMENDED DAILY ALLOWANCE

10 mg (12 to 600 IU)

3. SOURCES

- Wheat germ
- Alfalfa
- Green vegetables
- Safflower oil
- Eggs
- Walnuts, almonds, hazelnuts

VITAMIN E

- Sunflower seeds and oil
- Bananas, carrots, tomatoes

4. EFFECTS OF VITAMIN E DEFICIENCY

- Lusterless, dry hair
- Hair loss
- Prostate enlargement
- Gastro-intestinal problems
- Cardiovascular disorders
- Impotence
- Sterility
- Miscarriage
- Muscle deterioration

5. DESTROYED OR INHIBITED BY

- Rancid fats and oils
- Oral contraceptives
- High temperature
- Light
- Freezing

6. SPECIFIC APPLICATIONS

- Allergies
- Arthritis
- Arteriosclerosis

- Baldness
- Elevated cholesterol
- Cystitis
- Diabetes
- Angina
- Rheumatism
- Menstruation
- Menopause
- Migraines
- Headaches
- Obesity
- Phlebitis
- Sinusitis
- Stress
- Thrombosis
- Varicose veins
- Burns
- Scars
- Warts
- Wrinkles

7. NATURAL DIETARY SUPPLEMENTS

- Wheat-germ oil (capsules)
- Wheat-germ flakes
- Concentrated wheat-germ oil, Natural E (75 to 400 IU)

8. RECOMMENDATIONS

• If you freeze garden fruits and vegetables, remember that their vitamin E content will be significantly reduced.

• 100 g of white bread contains 0.23 mg of vitamin E, while the same amount of whole-wheat bread contains 1.3 mg.

• Polyunsaturated fats increase the body's need for vitamin E, so people who regularly eat margarine instead of butter need more vitamin E.

VITAMIN F

Non-saturated fatty acids
Fat-soluble
Consists of a group of polyunsaturated fatty acids, referred to as essential because the body cannot produce them
Principal essential fatty acids: linoleic acid, gamma-linolenic acid, arachidonic acid, and alpha-linolenic acid

1. FUNCTIONS

• Ensures the structure of cellular membranes
• Helps synthesize lecithin, myelin (insulates and nourishes nerve sheaths), and prostaglandins
Prostaglandins play a role in:
- Cardiovascular performance
- Muscle activity
- Intestinal secretion of water and electrolytes
- Stimulation of renal hormone secretions

2. RECOMMENDED DAILY ALLOWANCE

12 to 25 g

VITAMIN F

3. SOURCES

See section 7.

4. EFFECTS OF VITAMIN F DEFICIENCY

- Acne
- Diarrhea
- Allergies
- Dry skin
- Persistent thirst
- Gallstones
- Nail problems
- Nervous tension
- Dry, brittle hair
- Psoriasis
- Arteriosclerosis
- Myocardial infarction
- Angina

5. DESTROYED OR INHIBITED BY

- Radiation
- X-rays
- High temperatures
- Non-virgin oils that are not cold-pressed

6. SPECIFIC APPLICATIONS

- Allergies
- Baldness
- Asthma
- Elevated cholesterol or triglycerides
- Eczema
- Gall bladder
- Premature aging
- Menstrual cramps
- Varicose ulcers
- Psoriasis
- Overweight or underweight
- Nervous disorders
- Menopause problems
- Diabetes, cellulitis
- Diet imbalance
- Cancer
- Thrombosis
- Low immunity
- Arteriosclerosis
- Infertility
- Multiple sclerosis
- Gout
- Arthrosis
- Rheumatism
- Environmental pollution
- Medication and toxins
- Abdominal pain

VITAMIN F

7. NATURAL DIETARY SUPPLEMENTS

- Cold-pressed virgin sunflower oil–2 tbsp per day provides linolenic acid requirements
- Wheat-germ oil linolenic–1 tbsp occasionally
- Borage oil contains 16% to 23% gamma-linolenic acid
- Evening-primrose oil contains 6% to 10% gamma-linolenic acid
- Halibut-liver oil contains 10% to 20% eicosapentaenoic acid

8. RECOMMENDATIONS

- Therapeutic dosages of borage or evening-primrose oil, 2 or 3 times per year, are suggested for people whose daily diet does not include cold-pressed oils.
- Vitamin F is highly recommended for the elderly.

VITAMIN K

Phytomenadione
Fat-soluble

1. FUNCTIONS

Helps blood coagulation

2. RECOMMENDED DAILY ALLOWANCE

10 mcg (infant) to 140 mcg (maximum adult dose)

3. SOURCES

- Green, leafy vegetables
- Fruit
- Vegetable oils
- Goat's milk

4. EFFECTS OF VITAMIN K DEFICIENCY

- Diarrhea
- Increased tendency to hemorrhage
- Nose bleeds

VITAMIN K

5. DESTROYED OR INHIBITED BY

- Aspirin
- Excess antibiotics
- Radiation
- Rancid oil
- Sulfa drugs

6. SPECIFIC APPLICATIONS

- Contusions
- Hematomas
- Hemorrhaging
- Gall stones
- Irregular or painful menstruation
- Miscarriages

7. NATURAL DIETARY SUPPLEMENT

- Beef-liver capsules

8. RECOMMENDATION

- Vitamin K is recommended for heavy menstrual flow or cramps.

VITAMIN P

Also known as flavonoid or rutin
Blood-capillary vitamin
Water-soluble

1. FUNCTIONS

• Has coagulant properties similar to vitamins K and C
• Works synergistically with vitamins K and C

2. RECOMMENDED DAILY ALLOWANCE

80 to 100 mg

3. SOURCES

• Buckwheat
• Lettuce, oranges, lemons, apricots
• Almonds

4. EFFECTS OF VITAMIN P DEFICIENCY
• Hypertension
• Vascular problems
• Hemorrhaging
• Hematoma

VITAMIN P

5. DESTROYED OR INHIBITED BY

- Heat from cooking
- Tobacco
- Stress

6. SPECIFIC APPLICATIONS

- Weak capillaries and blood vessels
- Surgery
- Hemophilia
- Psoriasis
- Arteriosclerosis
- Varicose ulcers
- Hypertension
- Varicose veins
- Hemorrhoids
- Eczema

7. NATURAL DIETARY SUPPLEMENTS

- Supplements such as rose hips and acerola, which are rich in vitamin C, also contain a certain amount of vitamin P.

8. RECOMMENDATION

• Vitamin P therapy is recommended before surgery, and for people who tend to bruise or swell easily.

VITAMIN P

NATURAL VITAMIN SUPPLE- MENTS

1. HONEY

Bees produce honey from plant nectar and other sugary botanical solutions. The nectar is enriched within their bodies, then stored in honeycombs and allowed to ripen.

COMPOSITION

• The glucose and levulose–carbohydrates in honey are quickly assimilated by the body
• Diastases–molecules that ensure assimilation
• Organic acids
• Vitamins A, B, C, D, E, K
• Bactericides that act as antibiotic agents
• Proteins, pollen grains, and aromatic elements

The nutritional and therapeutic value of honey has been recognized through the ages. It is a healthy and natural product.

HONEY ENHANCES GOOD HEALTH BY PROVIDING:

• Increased resistance to physical and intellectual fatigue

HONEY

• An immediate source of energy for physical activity
• Moderation of vitamin deficiencies
• Laxative, antiseptic, sedative, and anti-toxic properties

I RECOMMEND HONEY FOR:

• Stomach and duodenal ulcers
• Intestinal infections
• Anemia
• Heart conditions
• Inflammation or infections of the mouth, nose, and throat
• Lung or bronchial problems (asthma, whooping cough, pneumonia, bronchitis, tuberculosis)

HONEY IS ALSO...

• A remarkable antitoxin, helpful in cases of alcohol or mushroom poisoning
• A diuretic that assists kidney function
• A sedative, particularly linden or orange-blossom honey
• A natural enhancer for the skin

2. POLLEN

Beekeepers say that pollen is the staff of life for bees, as it plays an essential role within the colony. Bees transport the pollen on their front legs, and an average hive has an annual pollen harvest of about 3 kg.

Pollen must be dried immediately, so that it is not altered or fermented. It may be eaten in its natural form, or mixed with honey to facilitate absorption.

POLLEN HAS AN ENRICHED COMPOSITION

- Approximately 35% protein (nitrogenous elements)
- Large amount of carbohydrates (40% sucrose)
- Low in fats
- Numerous vitamins: B_1, B_2, B_3, B_4, B_5, B_6, B_7, B_8, B_9, B_{12}, C, D, E, and provitamin A (beta-carotene)
- Rutin (helps strengthen capillaries)
- Enzymes
- Antibiotic constituents

BEES AND POLLEN

- Bees are excellent pollinating agents

POLLEN

- Because of its high protein content, pollen is reserved within the hive for feeding the larvae, providing them with the necessary elements for growth and development

POLLEN'S MAJOR CHARACTERISTICS

- Tonic and stimulant
- Restores functional equilibrium
- Detoxifies the body

FOR THOSE IN GOOD HEALTH

- Improves intellectual and physical performance
- Reinforces immunity against flu and other viral infections
- Helps overcome nutritional deficiencies during pregnancy and while breast-feeding

SPECIFIC APPLICATIONS

- Asthenia (general fatigue)
- Overexertion, convalescence or physical exhaustion
- Anorexia or loss of appetite
- Senescence (premature aging)
- Generalized weight loss
- Rickets or growth delay

EFFECT ON THE DIGESTIVE SYSTEM

- Stimulates gastric secretions
- Has laxative properties, but is not harmful to the intestines
- Helpful in cases of chronic diarrhea, as it regulates intestinal functions

GENERAL BENEFICIAL EFFECTS

- Cardiovascular system–for arteriosclerosis, arterial hypertension, and to strengthen capillaries
- Genito-urinary system–effective for cases of enlarged prostate, sexual impotence, and sexual asthenia

RECOMMENDED THERAPEUTIC TREATMENT

- For those in good health, treatment consists of one level tsp (5 g) daily, for three months.
- For people who are ill, therapeutic dosages may be as high as 2 tbsp (30 g) daily.

POLLEN

3. ROYAL JELLY

The development of a queen bee from an ordinary larva depends entirely on diet. The future queen is fed exclusively on royal jelly, while future worker bees receive this substance for only three days.

COMPOSITION-RICH AND COMPLEX

- 65% water
- 12—16% protein
- 9—10% carbohydrates (sugar)
- 5% lipids (fat)
- Amino acids essential for life (alanine, arginine, etc.)
- Vitamins (especially B-complex): A, B_1—B_{12}, C, D, E
- Calcium, iron, potassium, silicon, phosphorus, and other minerals
- Antibiotic properties

APPLICATIONS

- For those in good health, helps prevent vitamin, mineral, and amino-acid deficiencies
- Increases resistance and helps overcome physical and intellectual fatigue
- Improves appetite

• Can be included in weight-loss diets, as it is low in calories

• Beneficial general effect on the cardiovascular system, low blood pressure, and arteriosclerosis

• Beneficial for the genito-urinary system–sexual impotence and sexual asthenia are often remedied by a three-month therapeutic treatment

• Many neurasthenic and depressive states also respond well to treatment with royal jelly

• Late-autumn therapeutic treatment is useful, even though results are often not evident until the end of winter

ROYAL JELLY

4. WHEAT GERM

Wheat germ is the embryo of the wheat kernel and its most nutritious component.

Nature has endowed wheat germ with a number of valuable nutrients: carbohydrates, aromatic oils, proteins, minerals, hormones, and enzymes. It also contains essential vitamins: vitamin A (growth); vitamin B_1 (circulation); vitamin B_2 (metabolism); vitamins B_3 through B_6 (nerves); vitamin C (anti-scurvy); vitamin D (anti-rickets); vitamin E (fertility); vitamin F, etc.

Because of its nutritional value, wheat germ is included in athletes' diets, and should be taken by anyone who requires high physical endurance. It is also excellent for the skin.

Wheat germ can be purchased in health-food stores. It is available in flakes, oil, and capsules of various dosages.

5. SPIRULINA

Spirulina is a type of algae, harvested in Mexico, Hawaii, and a variety of other tropical areas. It is rich in vegetable protein and easily absorbed by the body.

AVERAGE VITAMIN CONTENT OF SPIRULINA

VITAMIN	mg/kg
Biotin (B_{17}, H)	0.4
Cyanocobalamin (B_{12})	0.4
Calcium pantothenate (B_5)	11.0
Folic acid	0.5
Inositol (B_7)	350.0
Nicotinic acid (B_3)	118.0
Pyridoxine (B_6)	3.0
Riboflavin (B_2)	40.0
Thiamin (B_1)	55.0
Tocopherol (E)	190.0
Beta-carotene (provitamin A)	2,500.0

SPIRULINA

Spirulina is significant because of the diversity of its B-complex vitamins. It is often recommended as a nutritional supplement to vegetarians, as their diet may be deficient in vitamin B_{12}.

Spirulina helps athletes assimilate vegetable protein more easily.

For people who are on a weight-loss diet, spirulina capsules can be taken as an appetite suppressant–three times daily, one hour before meals.

6. BREWER'S YEAST

Brewer's yeast is the best dietary supplement for B-complex vitamin deficiencies. It also contains valuable minerals (see chapter 8.)

TYPICAL COMPOSITION OF BREWER'S YEAST (PER 100 G)

Protein	46.00 g
Carbohydrates	36.00 g
Lipids (fats)	1.00 g
Vitamin B_1	12.00 mg
Vitamin B_2	4.00 mg
Vitamin B_3	1.40 mg
Vitamin B_5	33.00 mg
Vitamin B_6	4.00 mg
Vitamin B_9	0.04 mg
Vitamin B_{12}	0.02 mg
Biotin	0.11 mg
Choline	322.00 mg

BREWER'S YEAST

Therapeutic dosages of brewer's yeast may be taken every two months. If tablets are difficult to swallow, they can be dissolved in a glass of fruit juice.

Brewer's yeast is also recommended for pets, to improve the quality of their coats.

PART 2

MINERALS AND TRACE ELEMENTS

INTRODUCTION

In part one of this book, we discussed how indispensable vitamins are for good health. However, it is important not to overlook some other factors that are just as vital to our bodies: minerals and trace elements.

You are probably already aware of the existence of certain minerals, such as calcium, iron, fluoride, and phosphorus. However, you may not be familiar with the role they play in maintaining our bodies, the amounts we require daily, which foods are mineral-rich, or what can happen if we do not receive sufficient quantities. These topics will be dealt with in the remainder of this guide.

Minerals and trace elements are currently a matter of great interest, and knowing as much about them as possible can contribute to your good health.

MINERAL BASICS

Our metabolism depends upon our psychological and physical health. Due to the accelerated pace of modern life, we often find ourselves under a great deal of stress. Furthermore, our dietary intake is sometimes limited to fast foods or pre-packaged meals reheated in the microwave.

However, we should occasionally take time to examine our nutritional intake, as certain nutrients are indispensable for good health. These include water, carbohydrates, proteins, fats, vitamins, and minerals.

Most of the human body, 96%, is made up of four elements: oxygen (O), hydrogen (H), carbon (C), and nitrogen (N). The remaining 4% constitutes another group of approximately a hundred elements, without which life would be impossible.

Some of these are fairly well known: fluoride helps prevent cavities; iron is prescribed after severe blood loss; calcium supplements are suggested for pregnant women; and students should take phosphorus supplements before exams.

Thus, knowledge of the beneficial effects of certain minerals is not entirely new. We know that, along with vitamins, they help metabolize the nutrients required by the body. However, advanced research and observation of certain deficiencies have recently emphasized the significance of minerals and trace elements. Since they are essential for the body's metabolism, they should be carefully considered when we examine our daily nutritional intake.

5.

QUESTIONS ABOUT MINERALS AND TRACE ELEMENTS

1.

What are minerals?
Minerals are chemical elements found in mineral or crystalline states in nature. They are indispensable for metabolism, and are present in fairly significant quantities in the human body.

2.

What are trace elements?
Trace elements are also essential minerals, but they are required only in infinitesimal quantities. Since it is impossible for the body to synthesize trace elements, they must be included in our diet. Prolonged deficiencies can cause certain imbalances.

3.

What is the difference between them?
It is important to understand the difference between minerals and trace elements. The following examples may help illustrate their different roles.
A slice of bread with cheese eaten at breakfast contains glucides (carbohydrates) in the bread, plus lipids (fats) and calcium in the cheese. The calcium in the

cheese will contribute to the building of the body's bone structure.

The bread's glucides, referred to as complex carbohydrates, begin to be processed when mastication (chewing) separates the starch $C_6(H_{10}O_5)$ into smaller molecules. Good mastication should take about 20 seconds for each mouthful. The paste thus obtained travels to the stomach, where it is reduced by stomach secretions to a semi-liquid mass known as chyme, and the starch is broken down into small molecules of glucose $C_6H_{12}O_6$. These molecules, along with other elements, are then absorbed and assimilated by the intestinal villi, which are irrigated by the blood capillaries.

The glucose reaches the cellular level through the blood vessels. Each cell contains many organelles, which help the body maintain the balance necessary for good health. Mitochondria, for example, are the organelles that break down glucose.

In the mitochondria, the glucose undergoes hundreds of successive transformations, or biochemical reactions. When these reactions occur in the presence of oxygen (which is also carried by the blood vessels) they create respiration by-products: carbon dioxide (CO_2), water, and energy. This process is important for all living species.

The energy resulting from this process is very useful for the body's metabolism. An active person needs a considerable amount of energy to:

- maintain body temperature between 36.5° C and 37.5° C
- perform intellectual and physical tasks
- ensure proper functioning of the different organs (metabolism).

Chemical reactions take place in the body at a temperature of 37° C. At this relatively low temperature, these reactions need assistance in order to achieve their goals. Certain "helpers" are required to transform one molecule into another:

- the body chemicals
- enzymes (biochemical molecules that accelerate chemical reactions)
- trace elements such as gold, platinum, and silver.

Because trace elements are essential to certain biochemical reactions, a deficiency can cause imbalances in cellular tissues. This provides a fertile environment for the development of viruses and bacteria, and may lead to disease. Thousands of such occurrences can be found in all living species–plants, animals, and humans.

Another example of the difference between minerals and trace elements involves calcium. Calcium (in conjunction with phosphorus and magnesium) acts as a mineral when it helps the body's growth by building bones. However, as a 1% trace element, it performs a more subtle function at the cellular level.

4.

When were the beneficial roles of minerals and trace elements discovered?
The value of minerals has been recognized since the eighteenth century. However, the role of trace elements was not discovered until the end of the nineteenth century, with the advent of biochemistry. Research continues to produce interesting new information about these little-known elements.

5.

Do I have a deficiency or an excess?
Deficiencies of trace elements are difficult to detect. However, depending on the symptoms, doctors and therapists can often offer helpful advice.

By analyzing our nutritional intake, we may also note certain deficiencies. The test in chapter 6 can provide further useful information.

Today, some laboratories can test for various levels of trace elements, usually by analyzing blood, plasma, and hair. Diagnosis, however, must be done by a medical specialist.

6.

When should I start mineral therapy? How long should it last?

Therapy can help to re-establish the body's balance. The recommended duration of treatment is one month, three times per year. As always, it is advisable to consult your doctor or a dietitian before beginning treatment.

7.

How are minerals and trace elements used?

Minerals and trace elements are assimilated in combination with similar elements, and often with vitamins. You can find minerals and trace elements in drugstores and health-food stores. They are available in different forms:

• Chelated minerals (bio-available). These are bound to amino acids, for more efficient assimilation.

• Trace elements (alone or in complexes) in liquid form. The tincture is taken in the morning on an empty stomach. Consult your doctor about the dosage, which is usually between 15 and 30 drops, placed under the tongue using a plastic spoon.

8.

Minerals and modern life

As discussed in chapter 1, modern life can cause pathological fatigue in certain individuals. When this occurs, it emphasizes any natural imbalances in the body, and causes discomfort due to the loss of minerals and trace elements.

Agricultural practices have changed considerably over the last few decades. Intensive land use has resulted in an increase in production, but a decrease in quality. Overuse of chemical fertilizers saturates plant roots with too much of one substance, preventing the absorption of other necessary elements from the soil.

A similar nutritional process can block the body's absorption of essential minerals. For example, because of their tannin content, tea and red wine can slow the absorption of iron. Coffee interferes with the absorption of iron, potassium, and calcium. Alcohol produces a loss of zinc, copper, calcium, magnesium, and potassium.

Processing methods can also diminish the quantity of minerals. White bread may contain three times less magnesium than whole-grain bread. Green peas lose 33% of their mineral content when frozen, and as much as 42% when canned. When sugar is refined, it loses phosphorus, calcium, magnesium, iron, copper, zinc, fluoride, and manganese.

Certain medication combine with minerals, preventing their assimilation by the body:
- Diuretics drain potassium and magnesium
- Sedatives reduce the amount of calcium and magnesium in the blood
- Antacids, if taken in large quantities, prevent the assimilation of iron, and eliminate phosphorus through the urine
- Daily doses of aspirin remove between 1 and 2 mg of iron from the blood
- Cortico-steroids lower potassium levels, and cause calcium and magnesium to be eliminated through the urine.

Additives can also be detrimental to mineral absorption. For example, the phosphates used in soft drinks, ice cream, candy, beer, bread, and pastry combine with iron, preventing it from being assimilated by the blood. Other dangerous substances are also sometimes present in food; lead is detrimental to the brain, nerves, blood, and digestion; cadmium affects the lungs; and mercury affects coordination.

Finally, certain minerals can interact with others. An excess of sodium, for example, will eliminate calcium.

6.

THE EASY-CHEK® MINERAL-DEFICIENCY TEST

The reader is cautioned that the following evaluation test for requirements for specific minerals and trace elements is not intended to replace a blood test or professional medical advice.

There are many elements that cannot be included in this test, because not enough is yet known about them. These include aluminum, boron, silver, gold, strontium, mercury, titanium, and lithium, all of which contribute to the structure of life.

Classifications for the mineral-deficiency test are presented in alphabetical order. This should make it easier to complete the test and calculate your results.

HOW TO
COMPLETE THE TEST :

Circle the check-mark (✓) for the conditions and symptoms that apply to your particular case. For example, you may be a woman who smokes, practises sports, and lives in the city. You may also suffer from fatigue, arthritis, and insomnia, etc.

See page 130 to help analyze your test results.

CATEGORY	Calcium	Chromium	Cobalt	Copper	Fluoride
Child	✓				
Adult Female	✓				
Adult Male					
Urban dweller					
Athletic					
Takes oral contraceptives	✓			✓	
Smoker					
Uses alcohol	✓				
Drinks coffee	✓				
S Y M P T O M S					
Acne	✓				
Aging					
Allergies	✓				
Anemia			✓		
Anorexia					
Anxiety			✓		
Arteriosclerosis		✓			
Arthritis	✓			✓	
Asthenia (lack of body strength)					

Germanium	Iodine	Iron	Magnesium	Manganese	Molybdenum	Phosphorus	Potassium	Selenium	Silicon	Sodium	Sulphur	Zinc
		✓										
		✓						✓				
								✓				✓
		✓	✓					✓				
			✓			✓						
		✓										✓
								✓				✓
		✓	✓			✓	✓					✓
							✓					
	✓		✓				✓					✓
			✓					✓			✓	✓
			✓	✓			✓				✓	
		✓			✓							
		✓				✓				✓		✓
			✓									
	✓								✓		✓	✓
✓				✓		✓					✓	✓
				✓						✓		

SYMPTOMS	Calcium	Chromium	Cobalt	Copper	Fluoride
Asthma					
Baldness				✓	
Bruising (frequent)	✓				
Burns				✓	
Cancer					
Cardiac (heart attack)		✓		✓	
Cavities (dental)	✓				✓
Cholesterol		✓			
Cicatrization (slow healing)					
Colitis					
Concentration (lack of)					
Constipation					✓
Cramps (muscular)	✓				
Demineralization	✓				✓
Depression	✓				
Diabetes		✓			
Diarrhea			✓		
Digestive problems				✓	
Eczema	✓			✓	

Germanium	Iodine	Iron	Magnesium	Manganese	Molybdenum	Phosphorus	Potassium	Selenium	Silicon	Sodium	Sulphur	Zinc
	✓			✓								
												✓
		✓										
							✓		✓			
✓			✓					✓				
✓							✓	✓	✓			
			✓		✓	✓						
			✓									✓
			✓						✓		✓	
		✓	✓				✓					
		✓		✓		✓						✓
		✓	✓				✓					
			✓				✓			✓		
	✓		✓		✓				✓			
			✓									✓
			✓	✓			✓	✓				✓
							✓					
							✓					
	✓									✓		

SYMPTOMS	Calcium	Chromium	Cobalt	Copper	Fluoride
Eye problems					
Fatigue			✓		
Growth disorder	✓			✓	✓
Hypertension	✓	✓	✓		
Hypoglycemia		✓			
Immuno-defense system				✓	
Influenza					
Insomnia	✓				
Menstruation (painful)	✓				
Migraines	✓				
Muscles (sore)					
Nails (brittle)	✓				
Nervousness	✓				✓
Nervous disorders	✓		✓	✓	
Obesity	✓	✓			✓
Osteoporosis	✓				
Pregnancy	✓				
Prostate					
Psoriasis	✓				
Rickets	✓				✓

Germanium	Iodine	Iron	Magnesium	Manganese	Molybdenum	Phosphorus	Potassium	Selenium	Silicon	Sodium	Sulphur	Zinc
					✓							✓
		✓	✓	✓		✓	✓					✓
							✓		✓			
			✓					✓				
				✓			✓					
			✓	✓				✓			✓	✓
✓			✓									
			✓				✓					
		✓	✓									
			✓		✓			✓				
								✓				
		✓		✓				✓				✓
			✓				✓					
			✓	✓		✓			✓			
	✓		✓			✓		✓				
✓						✓						
			✓									
			✓								✓	
			✓					✓			✓	✓
			✓			✓			✓			

SYMPTOMS	Calcium	Chromium	Cobalt	Copper	Fluoride
Rheumatism	✓			✓	
Spasmophillia	✓		✓		
Stress	✓				
Skin disease				✓	
Skin (dry)					
Tetany (spasms)					
Tremors	✓				
Ulcers					
Varicose Veins	✓			✓	
Vomiting					
Wounds					
Wrinkles					
- - - - - - - -					
TOTAL OCCURRENCES - B	32	7	7	13	7
YOUR TOTAL - A					
YOUR PERCENTAGE SCORE : (A/B) X 100					

Germanium	Iodine	Iron	Magnesium	Manganese	Molybdenum	Phosphorus	Potassium	Selenium	Silicon	Sodium	Sulphur	Zinc
✓	✓		✓	✓				✓				✓
	✓					✓						
									✓		✓	
		✓					✓					✓
			✓			✓	✓					
			✓									
		✓	✓									
			✓									
					✓					✓		
									✓			✓
								✓				✓
6	9	16	36	12	6	12	20	14	12	6	8	24

CALCULATING AND UNDERSTANDING YOUR TEST RESULTS

1. Circle the check-marks that apply to you.

2. At the bottom of the last page of each column, enter the total number of check-marks circled for that column.

3. Divide <u>your</u> total, **A** in the chart, by the row **B** total (the total number of possible symptom occurrences for a particular mineral or trace element), then multiply the result by 100 to obtain a percentage.

3. Enter the percentage obtained for each column in the corresponding space.

ANALYSIS

0% to 35%: You are in good health, but should ensure that your diet is nutritionally balanced.

36% to 70%: It is time to pay more attention to your health. Try to include more mineral-rich foods in your diet, and consider taking supplements to replenish the minerals you are missing.

71% to 100%: You are suffering from serious mineral deficiencies, and should consult your physician.

Refer to the table in chapter 9.

7.

PROPERTIES OF MINERALS AND TRACE ELEMENTS

CALCIUM - CA

1. FUNCTIONS

- Almost all, 99%, of body calcium is used in the formation of bones and teeth; the remaining 1% regulates intercellular exchanges
- Growth factor (in conjunction with phosphorus)
- Important for muscular functioning (in conjunction with magnesium)
- Facilitates neural transmission, and is an essential supplement in cases of nervous breakdown
  Blood-coagulation agent
  Helps assimilate vitamin B_{12}

2. RECOMMENDED DAILY ALLOWANCE

800 to 2,000 mg

3. SOURCES

- Milk (1.1 g per litre)
- Cheese (Emmenthal: 1,080 mg per litre)
- Yogurt
- Beef liver (1 g per 500 g)
- Soybeans, watercress, cabbage
- Nettles and dandelion greens

CALCIUM

- Dried beans (137 mg per 100 g)
- Wheat germ
- Chocolate (100 mg per 100 g)
- Tofu
- Sesame seeds
- Hazelnuts (200 mg per 100 g)

4. EFFECTS OF CALCIUM DEFICIENCY

- Dental cavities
- Muscle cramps
- Menstrual cramps
- Numbness of limbs
- Insomnia
- Brittle nails
- Osteoporosis
- Palpitations

5. DESTROYED OR INHIBITED BY

- Stress
- Lack of exercise
- Overconsumption of alcohol or soft drinks
- Vitamin D deficiency
- Excessive consumption of eggs, chicken, or lamb
- Coffee and tea
- Rhubarb
- Oral contraceptives

6. SPECIFIC APPLICATIONS

- Arthritis
- Acne
- Allergies
- Backaches
- Breast-feeding
- Children
- Contraceptive pills
- Cramps in feet and legs
- Denture wearing
- Depression
- Eczema
- Fragile bones
- Gray hair
- Growth
- Hypertension
- Insomnia
- Menopause
- Migraines
- Nervousness
- Pregnancy
- Psoriasis
- Rheumatism
- Excess weight
- Tremors
- Tetany (muscle spasms)
- Varicose veins

CALCIUM

CALCIUM

7. NATURAL DIETARY SUPPLEMENTS

- Juices (horseradish, beet, potato, and tomato)
- CaPSi (capsules containing calcium, phosphorus, and silicon)
- Tofu (no cholesterol, rich in protein)

8. RECOMMENDATIONS

- The calcium/phosphorus ratio should be 1/1, generally speaking. It is higher for babies and lower for older people, who often have a deficiency of 30%.
- A balance of vitamins A, D, and C is necessary to keep calcium active and to allow its assimilation by the body. A pH balance is also required.
- The body eliminates between 200 and 300 mg of calcium daily through the urine and stools.
- People who wear dentures require more calcium.

CHROMIUM - CR

1. FUNCTIONS

• Found in insulin; regulates metabolism of carbohydrates

• Prevents cardiovascular disease by lowering blood cholesterol

• Helps regulate blood pressure

2. RECOMMENDED DAILY ALLOWANCE

50 to 300 mcg

3. SOURCES

• Brewer's yeast
• Natural whole-grain cereals
• Bran
• Black pepper, thyme, red peppers
• Mushrooms

4. EFFECTS OF CHROMIUM DEFICIENCY

• Arteriosclerosis
• Diabetes
• Hypoglycemia
• Glucose intolerance (diabetics)

CHROMIUM

5. D ESTROYED OR INHIBITED BY

- Excess sugar consumption
- Soft drinks, potato chips, cured meats (salami, pepperoni, etc.)

6. SPECIFIC APPLICATIONS

- Arteriosclerosis
- Blood circulation
- Couperose (skin-surface capillaries)
- Cardiac disorders
- Cholesterol
- Diabetes
- Hypertension
- Hypoglycemia
- Obesity
- Pregnancy
- Stress
- Triglycerides

7. NATURAL D IETARY SUPPLEMENTS

- Brewer's yeast (see chapter 8)
- Chromium drops (see chapter 7, section 7)

8. RECOMMENDATION

• People over 40 are susceptible to chromium deficiency. Pregnant women also need more chromium than usual.

CHROMIUM

COBALT - CO

1. FUNCTIONS

- An integral part of vitamin B_{12}
- Prevents anemia by renewing red-blood cells (200 million per minute)
- Regulates parasympathetic nervous system

2. RECOMMENDED DAILY ALLOWANCE

3 mcg

3. SOURCES

- Lentils
- Soy products
- Cherries, pears
- Milk

4. EFFECTS OF COBALT DEFICIENCY

- Anemia
- Anxiety
- Diarrhea
- Fatigue
- Hypertension

- Numbness of extremities
- Palpitations

5. DESTROYED OR INHIBITED BY

- Vitamin B_6 deficiency
- Iron deficiency

6. SPECIFIC APPLICATIONS

- Anemia
- Anxiety
- Cardiac arrythmia
- Diarrhea
- Fatigue
- Hypertension
- Numbness of extremities
- Pallid complexion

7. NATURAL DIETARY SUPPLEMENTS

- Vitamin B_{12}
- Spirulina (see chapter 4)
- Tamari

8. RECOMMENDATION
- Vegetarians should monitor their intake of cobalt through vitamin B_{12} regularly.

COPPER - CU

1. FUNCTIONS

- Assists in bone formation
- Participates in the production of red-blood-cell hemoglobin and maintains arterial flexibility
- Reinforces the immune system
- Constituent of myelin (covering for certain nerve fibres)
- Contributes to skin and hair pigmentation

2. RECOMMENDED DAILY ALLOWANCE

2 to 4 mg

3. SOURCES

- Walnuts, hazelnuts, almonds, apricots, chestnuts
- Molasses
- Black olives
- Watercress
- Vegetables
- Mushrooms
- Soybeans
- Algae

4. EFFECTS OF COPPER DEFICIENCY

- Arthritis
- Anemia
- Poor assimilation of iron
- General fatigue
- Skin diseases
- Lowered resistance to infection
- Cardiac problems

5. DESTROYED OR INHIBITED BY

- Excess zinc
- Pots and pans
- Water pipes
- Iron deficiency
- Oral contraceptives

6. SPECIFIC APPLICATIONS

- Anemia
- Baldness
- Burns
- Oral contraceptives
- Digestive problems
- Eczema
- Growth delay
- Low immunity

C
O
P
P
E
R

COPPER

- Rheumatism
- Varicose veins

7. NATURAL DIETARY SUPPLEMENTS

- Muesli
- Chelated copper capsules

8. RECOMMENDATIONS

- For inflammatory diseases such as rheumatism, wearing a copper bracelet is recommended.
- Wearing a copper bracelet for a few months also helps those who are sensitive to static electricity.

IRON - FE

1. FUNCTIONS

- Necessary for the production of red-blood-cell hemoglobin
- Gives the blood its red colour
- Stimulates the immune system and increases vitality
- Regulates metabolism of B-complex vitamins

2. RECOMMENDED DAILY ALLOWANCE

10 to 50 mg

3. SOURCES

- Beef liver (6—10 mg per 100 g)
- Egg yolks
- Fish
- Whole-grain cereals
- Soybeans (13 mg per 100 g)
- Parsley (18—23 mg per 100 g), spinach
- Walnuts, hazelnuts, almonds, figs, apricots, prunes, grapes
- Avocados

4. EFFECTS OF IRON DEFICIENCY

- Anemia
- Baldness
- Breathing difficulties
- Brittle nails
- Constipation
- Concentration problems
- Dry skin
- Hair loss
- General fatigue
- Loss of appetite
- Shortness of breath

5. DESTROYED OR INHIBITED BY

- Coffee, tea
- Excess zinc
- Phosphates (soft drinks, food additives)
- Copper deficiency
- Advanced age
- Oxalic acid, found in rhubarb and sorrel
- Excessive consumption of eggs
- Oral contraceptives

6. SPECIFIC APPLICATIONS

- Alcoholism

- Anemia
- Children
- Urban environment
- Colitis
- Constipation
- Oral contraceptives
- Frequent hemorrhaging
- Hemorrhoids
- Memory loss
- Menstrual problems
- Ulcers

7. NATURAL DIETARY SUPPLEMENTS

- Whole blueberry leaves (provide iron in the form of Fe_2+)
- Sauerkraut juice
- Beef-liver capsules
- Chelated-iron capsules

8. RECOMMENDATIONS

The human body contains 4 g of iron, 70% of which is found in the hemoglobin. Only 8% of all iron consumed can be assimilated, and this must occur in conjunction with vitamin B_{12} (cobalt), copper, manganese, and vitamin C. Therefore, iron supplements are required by:

- People who suffer from chronic fatigue, anemia, anxiety, constipation, or asthma
- Vegetarians, people on a weight-loss diet, and those recovering from surgery

IRON

FLUORIDE - F

1. FUNCTION

• Aids calcium assimilation and helps fight dental cavities.

2. RECOMMENDED DAILY ALLOWANCE

1 mg

3. SOURCES

• Fish
• Algae
• Sprouted grains
• Tea
• Dandelion greens, green cabbage, spinach

4. EFFECTS OF FLUORIDE DEFICIENCY

• Dental cavities
• Bone and vertebra deformities (scoliosis)
• Osteoporosis
• Rickets

FLUORIDE

5. DESTROYED OR INHIBITED BY

- Excess sugar consumption

6. SPECIFIC APPLICATIONS

- Growth disorders
- Osteoporosis
- Rickets
- Scoliosis

7. NATURAL DIETARY SUPPLEMENTS

- Fluoride drops
- Spirulina (see chapter 4)

8. RECOMMENDATIONS

- Do not exceed recommended dosage.
- Because fluoride has received so much publicity, many people are confused about its usage. If you are unsure, seek the advice of a physician or dietitian.

GERMANIUM - G

1. FUNCTIONS

- Reinforces the immune system
- An anti-oxidant for amino acids
- Contributes to healthy cell membranes

2. RECOMMENDED DAILY ALLOWANCE

50 to 100 mg

3. SOURCES

- Garlic
- Ginseng
- Mushrooms
- Comfrey

4. EFFECTS OF GERMANIUM DEFICIENCY

- Lowered immunity
- Disorders of the nervous system

GERMANIUM

5. DESTROYED OR INHIBITED BY

- Stress
- Alcohol
- Tobacco

6. SPECIFIC APPLICATIONS

- AIDS
- Arthritis
- Cancer
- Cardiovascular disease
- Coronary thrombosis
- Gastritis
- Hypertension
- Leukemia
- Myopathy (muscle-tissue disorder)
- Neural and endocrinological disorders
- Osteoporosis
- Parkinson's disease
- Rheumatism
- Multiple sclerosis
- Ulcers
- Viral infections

7. NATURAL DIETARY SUPPLEMENTS

- Bio-germanium capsules

- Ginseng (see chapter 4)

8. RECOMMENDATION

- Include garlic in your daily diet.

GERMANIUM

IODINE - I

1. FUNCTIONS

- Acts on the thyroid, regulating metabolism of protein, glucides, and lipids
- Participates in energy production
- Assists physical and mental development

2. RECOMMENDED DAILY ALLOWANCE

100 to 1,000 mcg

3. SOURCES

- Seafood
- Milk
- Algae
- Onions, radishes, mushrooms, turnips, green beans
- Prunes, gooseberries, blackberries
- Sea salt

4. EFFECTS OF IODINE DEFICIENCY

- Cold hands and feet
- Constipation

- Dry hair
- Irritability
- Nervousness
- Obesity

5. DESTROYED OR INHIBITED BY

- Stress

6. SPECIFIC APPLICATIONS

- Arteriosclerosis
- Asthma
- Cellulitis
- High cholesterol
- Loss of minerals
- Goitre
- Hair problems
- Hyperthyroidism
- Hypertension
- Obesity
- Overexertion
- Rheumatism (chronic)
- Premature aging

7. NATURAL DIETARY SUPPLEMENTS

- Milt (fish-sperm fluid)

IODINE

- Iodine capsules
- Algae capsules

8. RECOMMENDATIONS

Because the stress of modern life accelerates the aging process, people over forty are advised to take iodine supplements.

IODINE

MAGNESIUM - MG

1. FUNCTIONS

- Helps maintain balance of basic acids
- Helps metabolize blood sugar, calcium, and vitamin C
- Participates in DNA and RNA synthesis
- Muscle relaxant
- Regulates neural transmissions (anti-stress)
- Some studies show influence on tumour development

2. RECOMMENDED DAILY ALLOWANCE

300 to 350 mg

3. SOURCES

- Seafood
- Gruyère cheese (45 mg per 100 g)
- Wheat germ
- Natural whole-grain cereals and whole-wheat bread
- Onions, soy products, spinach
- Walnuts, hazelnuts, almonds (250 mg per 100 g)
- Sesame seeds

MAGNESIUM

4. EFFECTS OF MAGNESIUM DEFICIENCY

- Anxiety
- Confusion
- Cramps
- Delayed childhood development
- Headaches
- Insomnia
- Irritability
- Palpitations
- Tremors
- Spasmophillia

5. DESTROYED OR INHIBITED BY

- Excess calcium and phosphorus
- Excess vegetable consumption
- Alcohol
- Oral contraceptives
- Prolonged cooking
- Obesity
- Stress
- Cold temperatures

6. SPECIFIC APPLICATIONS

- Acne
- Premature aging
- Alcoholism

- Allergies
- Apathy
- Bruises (frequent)
- Cancer
- High cholesterol
- Constipation
- Cramps
- Dental cavities
- Depression
- Diabetes
- Excess body weight
- Fatigue
- Growth delay
- Headaches
- Hypertension
- Insect stings and bites
- Insomnia
- Kidney stones
- Urban environment
- Heavy manual labour
- Nervousness
- Pregnancy
- Premenstrual syndrome
- Prostate problems
- Psoriasis
- Relaxation of cardiac muscle
- Rheumatism
- Strenuous athletic exercise
- Stress

MAGNESIUM

MAGNESIUM

- Tetany
- Varicose veins

7. NATURAL DIETARY SUPPLEMENTS

- Horseradish and potato juices
- Quinton's Serum (sea water)
- Complete sea salt

8. RECOMMENDATIONS

- Ensuring daily magnesium intake is strongly recommended for those who drink alcohol, and for women taking oral contraceptives.
- Therapeutic dosages of magnesium are recommended for 15 days after insect stings or bites.
- Cats and dogs get the magnesium they need by eating grass.
- Magnesium is to plant chlorophyll what iron is to red-blood-cell hemoglobin.

MANGANESE - MN

1. FUNCTIONS

- Universal anti-allergenic
- Participates in the metabolism of vitamin B_1, glucides, and vitamin E
- Assists in sexual-hormone production
- Helps activate enzymes

2. RECOMMENDED DAILY ALLOWANCE

1 to 50 mg

3. SOURCES

- Egg yolks
- Liver
- Green leafy vegetables
- Natural whole-grain cereals
- Soy products
- Beets
- Raspberries, blueberries, pineapples, bananas
- Walnuts, hazelnuts

MANGANESE

4. EFFECTS OF MANGANESE DEFICIENCY

- Allergies
- Arthritis
- Ringing in the ears
- Hearing loss
- Nervous irritability
- Memory loss
- Morning fatigue

5. DESTROYED OR INHIBITED BY

- Calcium
- Excess phosphorus

6. SPECIFIC APPLICATIONS

- Allergies
- Asthma
- Asthenia
- Arthritis
- Ringing in the ears
- Diabetes
- Epilepsy
- Fatigue
- Low immunity
- Memory loss
- Poor muscle reflexes

7. NATURAL DIETARY SUPPLEMENTS

- Sauerkraut juice
- Manganese drops
- Bee pollen

8. RECOMMENDATIONS

- Allergy sufferers should increase their manganese intake.

MANGANESE

MOLYBDENUM - MO

1. FUNCTIONS

- Eliminates cellular toxins through the kidneys
- Helps assimilate iron and copper
- Enhances the effect of fluoride

2. RECOMMENDED DAILY ALLOWANCE

50 to 500 mcg

3. SOURCES

- Meat
- Natural whole-grain cereals
- Soybeans, spinach
- Yeast

4. EFFECTS OF MOLYBDENUM DEFICIENCY

- Dental cavities
- Headaches
- Nausea and vomiting
- Increased heart rate

• Vision problems

5. DESTROYED OR INHIBITED BY

Excess sugar

6. SPECIFIC APPLICATIONS

• Anemia
• Dental cavities
• Migraines
• Nausea
• Tachycardia
• Vomiting

7. NATURAL DIETARY SUPPLEMENTS

• Brewer's yeast (see chapters 4 and 10)

8. RECOMMENDATION

• Natural foods are preferable to processed foods, as they contain more molybdenum and other valuable minerals.

MOLYBDENUM

PHOSPHORUS - P

1. FUNCTIONS

• The body contains about 700 g of phosphorus: 80% in the bones, 10% in muscle tissue, and 10% in other tissues
• Required by the nervous system; one of the components of lecithin
• Produces chemical energy for the breakdown of carbohydrates (see chapter 1, section 3)
• Participates in the metabolism of calcium, glucides, lipids, and proteins
• Aids cellular growth and repair
• Facilitates the assimilation of vitamins

2. RECOMMENDED DAILY ALLOWANCE

800 to 1,500 mg (depending on age)

3. SOURCES

• Egg yolks (560 mg per 100 g)
• Cheese (gruyère: 600 mg per 100 g)
• Fish
• Poultry
• Sprouted soybeans (580 mg per 100 g)

- Natural whole grains (wheat germ: 1,200 mg per 100 g)
- Brewer's yeast (1,900 mg per 100 g)
- Almonds (470 mg per 100 g)

4. EFFECTS OF PHOSPHORUS DEFICIENCY

- Arthritis
- Loss of bone calcium
- Dental cavities
- Fatigue
- Gingivitis
- Inadequate kidney function
- Irregular respiration
- Loss of appetite
- Nervous disorders
- Rickets
- Weight loss

5. DESTROYED OR INHIBITED BY

- Aluminum
- Iron
- Excess magnesium
- Refined sugar
- Diuretics

PHOSPHORUS

6. SPECIFIC APPLICATIONS

- Arthritis
- Chronic alcoholism
- Convalescence
- Growth disorders
- Lack of appetite
- Mental stress
- Osteoporosis
- Obesity
- Rickets
- Spasmophilia
- Dental cavities and gum disease
- Excess uric acid

7. NATURAL DIETARY SUPPLEMENTS

- Potato and tomato juices
- Brewer's yeast
- Soya lecithin
- Bee pollen

8. RECOMMENDATIONS

- Meat, eggs, and fish are rich in phosphorus but deficient in calcium, as are soft drinks.

• Phosphate additives are used in preserved meats (salami, smoked meat) and in commercial bakery goods.

• Natural whole-grain bread is preferable to commercial bread, in which the phytic acid in yeast is not transformed into more usable phytates.

PHOSPHORUS

POTASSIUM - K

1. FUNCTIONS

• Nerve tranquilizer
• Assists muscular contraction (particularly the heart muscle) and neural transmission
• Improves kidney function to eliminate blood toxins
• Regulates quantity of trace minerals in cells

2. RECOMMENDED DAILY ALLOWANCE

100 to 300 mg

3. SOURCES

• Milk and cheese
• Tofu
• Apples, oranges, grapes
• Dates, figs, peaches, peanuts, chestnuts
• Blackstrap molasses
• Sunflower seeds
• Tomato juice
• Algae

4. EFFECTS OF POTASSIUM DEFICIENCY

- Acne
- Constipation
- Digestive problems
- Dry skin
- General weakness
- Hypertension
- Insomnia
- Mental and physical fatigue
- Nervousness
- Persistent thirst
- Weak reflexes

5. DESTROYED OR INHIBITED BY

- Alcohol
- Coffee
- Stress
- Cortisone, diuretics, laxatives, antibiotics
- Excess salt and sugar
- Diarrhea

6. SPECIFIC APPLICATIONS

- Acne
- Alcoholism
- Allergies

POTASSIUM

POTASSIUM

- Burns
- Cardiovascular disease
- Coffee
- Colic
- Cramps
- Diarrhea
- Diabetes
- Fatigue
- Growth disorders
- Hypertension

7. NATURAL DIETARY SUPPLEMENTS

- Wheat germ
- Bee pollen
- Algae
- Horseradish; beet, potato, and tomato juices

8. RECOMMENDATIONS

- The relationship between sodium and potassium is important at the cellular level.
- Natural organic foods are richer in potassium than in sodium.
- Athletes need more potassium, as well as more sodium, magnesium, zinc, and manganese.
- Potassium makes vegetables firmer and more pest-resistant.

SELENIUM - SE

1. FUNCTIONS

- As an anti-oxidant, fortifies the immune system
- Slows aging and prevents cardiovascular disease
- Reduces the effects of alcohol, tobacco, coffee, and pollution
- Acts in conjunction with vitamin C

2. RECOMMENDED DAILY ALLOWANCE

50 to 200 mcg (must not exceed 500 mcg)

3. SOURCES

- Seafood
- Whole-grain cereals, wheat germ
- Onions, tomatoes, broccoli
- Pineapple
- Brazil nuts
- Yeast

4. EFFECTS OF SELENIUM DEFICIENCY

- Decreased resistance to infection
- Muscular pain

SELENIUM

- Premature aging

5. DESTROYED OR INHIBITED BY

- Excess lipids (fats)
- Excess glucides (sugar)

6. SPECIFIC APPLICATIONS

- Couperose (broken surface capillaries)
- Cardiovascular disease
- Canned and frozen food
- Cancer
- Urban environment
- Dandruff
- Fertility
- Hypertension
- Men
- Older people
- Premature wrinkles
- Protection against pollution
- Psoriasis
- Rheumatism
- Tobacco

7. NATURAL DIETARY SUPPLEMENT

• In capsule form, selenium is most often combined with vitamin E.

8. RECOMMENDATION

• Selenium supplements are recommended for people over 30 at the rate of 100 mcg per day for 10 days of each month.

SELENIUM

SILICON - SI

1. FUNCTIONS

- Helps heal and replenish bone and skin tissue
- Prevents premature aging
- Necessary for healthy heart (aorta)
- Helps assimilate calcium, phosphorus, and magnesium

2. RECOMMENDED DAILY ALLOWANCE

20 to 30 mg

3. SOURCES

- Soybeans
- Alfalfa sprouts
- Fruit skins (from organically grown fruits)
- Natural whole grain cereals
- Onions, shallots, garlic, asparagus, radishes, cauliflower
- Horsetail

4. EFFECTS OF SILICON DEFICIENCY

- Poor healing

- Frequent fractures
- Brittle nails and hair

5. DESTROYED OR INHIBITED BY

- Pesticides and preservatives used on fresh fruit

6. SPECIFIC APPLICATIONS

- Arteriosclerosis
- Burns
- Dry, brittle hair
- Cancer
- Cellulitis
- Diabetes
- Growth disorders
- Heart attack
- Incomplete or poor healing of injuries

7. NATURAL DIETARY SUPPLEMENTS

- Alfalfa sprouts
- Horsetail capsules

8. RECOMMENDATIONS

- A diet that includes natural whole-grain cereals is rich in silicon.

SILICON

- Eat fruit skins whenever possible, as peeled fruit has no silicon.

SILICON

SODIUM - NA

1. FUNCTIONS

- Aids neural transmission to muscle fibres
- Related to water retention in kidneys

2. RECOMMENDED DAILY ALLOWANCE

300 mg

3. SOURCES

- Seafood
- Milk and cheese
- All meat products
- Sea salt

4. EFFECTS OF SODIUM DEFICIENCY

- Asthenia
- Cramps
- Intestinal gas
- Loss of appetite
- Mental difficulties
- Vomiting
- Weight loss

Sodium deficiency is very rare. An excess is much more common, and leads to hypertension.

SODIUM

5. DESTROYED OR INHIBITED BY

- Potassium deficiency
- Abuse of laxatives and diuretics

6. SPECIFIC APPLICATIONS

- Dehydration
- Dental arthritis
- Fever
- Oral infections
- Sore throat

7. NATURAL DIETARY SUPPLEMENTS

- Horseradish and potato juices
- Quinton's Serum
- Sea salt

8. RECOMMENDATIONS

- The required daily sodium intake is 5 g. However, the average daily intake is much higher–closer to 25 to 30 g. This excess can lead to hypertension and arteriosclerosis.
- People who smoke and drink alcohol require more sodium.

SULPHUR - S

1. FUNCTIONS

- Participates in collagen synthesis
- Aids tissue formation, ameliorates skin disease
- Anti-allergenic
- Improves liver and gall-bladder function (detoxicant)
- Included in the basic composition of many important molecules: amino acids, insulin, enzymes, antibodies, etc.

2. RECOMMENDED DAILY ALLOWANCE

Varies widely. Consult your physician.

3. SOURCES

- Whole milk, cream
- Fish
- Eggs
- Cheese
- Wheat germ
- Walnuts
- Black radish
- Garlic

SULPHUR

4. EFFECTS OF SULPHUR DEFICIENCY

- Allergies
- Dermatosis
- Eczema
- Liver and gall bladder problems
- Nettle rash, hives

5. DESTROYED OR INHIBITED BY

- Copper and manganese deficiencies

6. SPECIFIC APPLICATIONS

- Premature aging
- Arthritis
- Acne
- Allergies
- Chronic bronchitis
- Eczema
- Laryngitis
- Throat inflammation
- Psoriasis

7. NATURAL DIETARY SUPPLEMENTS

- Brewer's yeast

- Wheat germ
- Bee pollen
- Algae
- Sauerkraut and potato juices

8. RECOMMENDATIONS

- Sulphur soap can be used for skin infections–and it is also a good anti-perspirant.

S U L P H U R

ZINC -ZN

1. FUNCTIONS

• Helps activate enzymes, regulates phosphorus and protein metabolism
• Facilitates glucide digestion
• Important for growth and development of reproductive organs
• Hastens healing of wounds and burns
• Enhances night vision, taste, and smell

2. RECOMMENDED DAILY ALLOWANCE

15 to 100 mg

3. SOURCES

• Cheese
• Liver
• Cereals and sprouted grains
• Sunflower seeds
• Brewer's yeast
• Mushrooms, spinach
• Soybeans

4. EFFECTS OF ZINC DEFICIENCY

- Anorexia
- Inability to assimilate folic acid (vitamin B9)
- Fatigue
- Growth delay
- Loss of sense of taste
- Low resistance to infection
- Male sterility
- Rough skin
- Delayed sexual development
- White spots on fingernails

5. DESTROYED OR INHIBITED BY

- Tobacco (cadmium residue from smoke remains in the testicles)
- Alcohol
- Oral contraceptives
- Cortisone and cortisone derivatives
- Excess calcium
- Phosphorus deficiency
- Excess perspiration (strenuous labour or exercise)

6. SPECIFIC APPLICATIONS

- Acne
- Alcoholism

ZINC

- Arteriosclerosis
- Arthritis
- Baldness
- Brittle nails
- High cholesterol
- Cirrhosis
- Oral Contraceptives
- Diabetes
- Dry skin
- Headaches
- Healing wounds and burns
- Loss of smell
- Loss of taste
- Men
- Memory loss
- Migraines
- People taking cortisone
- Prostate problems
- Premature wrinkles
- Psoriasis
- Smokers
- Sun stroke
- Surgery
- Vegetarians
- Weak vision
- White spots on nails

7. NATURAL DIETARY SUPPLEMENTS

- Ginseng (see chapter 8)
- Beef-liver capsules

8. RECOMMENDATIONS

- Liver is an excellent dietary source of zinc. It also contains iron, copper, and potassium, making it an ideal antidote to modern stress.
- Zinc protects against lead emissions from automobiles, and against mosquito bites.
- Over-cultivation decreases the zinc content of soil.

8.
NATURAL MINERAL
SUPPLEMENTS

1. GINSENG

A perennial herb of the araliceae family, genus panax, the ginseng root has been called "the root of life." It has a long reputation as a panacea for a variety of ailments, including cancer, rheumatism, diabetes, sexual impotence, and aging. Soviet scientists have claimed that certain substances in ginseng stimulate endocrine secretions and act as a tonic to the cardio-vascular system.

COMPOSITION

- Glycosides
- Fat-soluble elements
- Vitamins A, B1, C, D, and B12
- Amino acids
- Phosphorus, potassium, calcium, magnesium, iron, germanium, sodium, zinc, copper, molybdenum, manganese, and boron

Ginseng also has an ancient reputation as an aphrodisiac. Today, it is recognized as an excellent food supplement. It contains many active ingredients vital for maintaining good health, and the advised therapeutic dosage is at least 1 gram per day.

GINSENG

Ginseng is particularly recommended for athletes, students studying for exams, convalescents, and the elderly. It also helps counteract the effects of stress, pollution, and nicotine.

Ginseng fortifies the liver, spleen, lungs, kidneys, and stomach. It fights fatigue and lack of appetite, and has tonic and calming properties for the nervous system.

Ginseng is available in many forms: capsules, powder, pure extract, or diluted in tonics. The best ginseng, aged for at least five years, is Korean.

2. CLAY

Clay is a remarkable substance, extremely rich in minerals. It is waterproof rock, containing particles that make it valuable for internal and external treatment, and is highly recommended. To learn about the health benefits of clay, an excellent source is the translation of Raymond Dextreit's book *L'argile qui guérit.*

COMPOSITION OF CLAY (G PER 100 G)

	White	Green	Blue
Silicon	51.10	48.25	63.00
Aluminum	32.90	11.17	31.60
Titanium	1.50	0.43	0.55
Iron	1.50	0.51	4.60
Sodium	0.10	0.50	0.68
Calcium	0.20	0.44	0.45
Magnesium	0.10	9.66	1.90
Potassium	0.40	3.03	1.88

Clay has many properties: stimulant, antiseptic, healer, cleanser, mineral replacement, and sedative. When preparing clay, do not heat it, do not use ordinary tap water, and avoid contact with metal or plastic utensils.

3. ALGAE

Algae are very rich in minerals and trace elements. In Japan, average consumption of algae is about 80 grams per day.

COMPOSITION

The average composition of algae includes potassium, magnesium, iodine, iron, copper, manganese, aluminum, selenium, zinc, silicon, and fluoride.

4. BREWER'S YEAST

In chapter 4, we discussed the vitamin content of brewer's yeast. In this section, we will consider its mineral content.

Brewer's yeast should be included in your regular diet. It is rich in minerals (which make up 7% to 8.5% of its contents), vitamins, and amino acids.

TYPICAL MINERAL COMPOSITION OF BREWER'S YEAST

Iron	75 ppm
Manganese	10 ppm
Copper	10 ppm
Zinc	40 ppm
Selenium	0.5 ppm
Phosphorus	1.2%
Potassium	1.6%
Calcium	0.2%
Iodides	4.0%

5. SEA SALT

Research has established consumption levels for sodium chloride (NaCl), or white salt. For instance, in European countries such as Belgium, daily consumption is 15 grams; in the United States, it is 18 grams. Such high consumption leads to greater risk of cardiovascular disease, as the average salt requirement is only 3—5 grams.

Sea salt is more beneficial than regular white salt because it offers a larger variety of minerals.

COMPOSITION OF SEA SALT (IN %)

Sodium	34.3	Carbon	0.07
Chlorine	53.7	Iron	0.014
Sulphur	1.16	Fluoride	0.00082
Magnesium	0.64	Phosphorus	0.00046
Calcium	0.23	Bromine	0.00025
Nitrogen	0.16	Iodine	0.0000112
Silicon	0.11		

This table represents an average analysis of unrefined sea salt. Sea salt also contains approximately twenty trace elements.

6. OTHER SOURCES

The following foods are also rich in mineral content:

A. COFFEE WITH MILK

Manganese, iron, zinc, copper, and rubidium

B. BEEF LIVER

Zinc, copper, iron, selenium, chromium, cobalt, potassium, and manganese

C. HONEY

Calcium, sodium, potassium, sulphur, magnesium, iodine, and iron

D. BEE POLLEN

Calcium, magnesium, potassium, phosphorus, silicon, and manganese

E. ROYAL JELLY

Calcium, iron, potassium, silicon, and phosphorus

9

VITAMIN & MINERAL RECAP TABLE

NAME	DESCRIPTION
Vitamin A	Growth, sight and skin vitamin
Vitamin B$_1$	Nervous and circulatory systems vitamin
Vitamin B$_2$	Energy and anti-muscle cramp vitamin
Vitamin B$_3$	High-energy vitamin
Vitamin B$_5$	Skin and hair vitamin
Vitamin B$_6$	Meat-eaters' vitamin
Vitamin B$_7$	Anti-anemia vitamin
Vitamin B$_9$	Anti-dermatosis vitamin
Vitamin B$_{12}$	Red blood-cell vitamin
Vitamin B$_{15}$	Vitamin for athletes
Vitamin B$_{17}$	Skin and hair vitamin
Choline	
Vitamin C	Anti-cold vitamin
Vitamin D	Bone vitamin
Vitamin E	Muscle and reproduction vitamin
Vitamin F	Modern life vitamin
Vitamin K	Blood coagulation vitamin
Vitamin P	Blood vessel vitamin

NAME	DESCRIPTION
Vitamin A	Growth, sight and skin vitamin
Vitamin B$_1$	Nervous and circulatory systems vitamin
Vitamin B$_2$	Energy and anti-muscle cramp vitamin
Vitamin B$_3$	High-energy vitamin
Vitamin B$_5$	Skin and hair vitamin
Vitamin B$_6$	Meat-eaters' vitamin
Vitamin B$_7$	Anti-anemia vitamin
Vitamin B$_9$	Anti-dermatosis vitamin
Vitamin B$_{12}$	Red blood-cell vitamin
Vitamin B$_{15}$	Vitamin for athletes
Vitamin B$_{17}$	Skin and hair vitamin
Choline	
Vitamin C	Anti-cold vitamin
Vitamin D	Bone vitamin
Vitamin E	Muscle and reproduction vitamin
Vitamin F	Modern life vitamin
Vitamin K	Blood coagulation vitamin
Vitamin P	Blood vessel vitamin

DAILY DOSE	NATURAL DIETARY SUPPLEMENTS
0.5 to 1.8 mg	Carrot oil or halibut oil capsules, provitamin, pollen
1 to 2 mg	Brewer's yeast
1.5 to 2.5 mg	Brewer's yeast
10 to 20 mg	Brewer's yeast
6 to 10 mg	Royal jelly capsules or pure, fresh royal jelly
2 mg	Brewer's yeast
100 mg	Brewer's yeast
0.01 to 0.4 mg	Brewer's yeast
10 mg	Brewer's yeast
3 mcg	Spirulina gelcaps
50 to 150 mg	Brewer's yeast
0.3 mg	Brewer's yeast
100 mg	
60 mg to 5 g	Rose-hip and acerola capsules
0.010 mg	Halibut liver oil capsules
10 mg	Wheat germ oil capsules
12 to 25 g	Evening-primrose or borage oil capsules
3-4 mg	Beef liver capsules
80-100 mg	Rose-hip and acerola capsules

ELEMENT OR SALT	SYMBOL	ROLES
Calcium	Ca	Bone/tooth formation - intercellular exchange
Chromium	Cr	Glucide metabolism-inhibits cardiovascular disease
Cobalt	Co	Regulates autonomic nervous system / Participates in red blood cell regeneration
Copper	Cu	Reinforces immune system
Fluoride	F	'Fixes' minerals and inhibits tooth decay
Germanium	Ge	Reinforces immune system and helps protect against effects of heavy metals
Iodine	I	Helps to regulate glucide, lipid and protein metabolism and acts on the thyroid gland
Iron	Fe	Hemoglobulin production agent/ Vitamin B group metabolism
Magnesium	Mg	Anti-stress/Glucide metabolism
Manganese	Mn	Antiallergenic, sexual hormone production chain
Molybdenum	Mo	Toxin reducer
Phosphorus	P	Glucide, lipid, protein, vitamin,mineral salt metabolism
Potassium	K	Toxin reducer/Mineral salt and trace element metabolizer
Selenium	Se	Antioxidant, immune system enhancer
Silicon	Si	Ant-aging
Sodium	Na	Essentiel for nervous system and kidneys
Sulphur	S	Antiallergenic/liver detoxication
Zinc	Zn	Protein/Phosphorus metabolism, healing, senses

DAILY DOSE	NATURAL DIETARY SUPPLEMENTS
800 to 2000 mg	Tofu, Calcium gelcaps
50 to 300 mcg	Brewer's yeast
3 mcg	Vitamin B_{12}
2 to 4 mg	Muesli
10 to 50 mg	Iron gelcaps
1 mg	Spirulina, Fluoride drops
50 to 100 mg	Ginseng, Biogermanium
100 to 1000 mcg	Fish milt
300 to 350 mg	Sea salt
1 to 50 mg	Pollen, manganese drops
50 to 500 mcg	Yeast
800 to 1500 mg	Yeast, lecithin
100 to 300 mg	Wheat germ, pollen, algae
50 to 200 mcg	Vitamin E and capsules
2 to 30 mg	Horsetail capsules
300 mg	Sea salt
Consult your doctor	Yeast, pollen, algae
15 to 100 mg	Ginseng, beef liver capsules

10.

INDEX OF HEALTH PROBLEMS AND VITAMIN/ MINERAL DEFICIENCIES

CONDITION	POSSIBLE VITAMIN/ MINERAL DEFICIENCY
Acne	Vitamins A, B6, D, F, iodine, potassium, zinc, calcium, magnesium
Aging	Vitamins B15, F, magnesium, selenium, sulphur, zinc
Alcoholism	Vitamins A, D, calcium, iron, magnesium, phosphorus, potassium, zinc
Allergies	Vitamins A, D, E, F, magnesium, manganese, potassium, sulphur, calcium
AIDS	Germanium
Anemia	Vitamin B9, cobalt, copper, iron, molybdenum
Angina	Vitamins E, F
Anorexia	Vitamin B1, iron, phosphorus, sodium, zinc
Anxiety	Vitamin B3, cobalt, magnesium
Apathy	Vitamin B6, magnesium
Appetite, lack of	Vitamins B3, B12, B9, B17

Arteriosclerosis	Vitamins E, F, chromium, iodine, silicon, sulphur, zinc
Arthritis	Vitamins A, D, E, calcium, copper, germanium, manganese, phosphorus, sulphur, zinc
Arthrosis	Vitamin F
Asthenia	Sodium, manganese
Asthma	Vitamins A, F, iodine, manganese
Backache	Calcium
Baldness	Copper, zinc
Bones, fragile	Calcium
Breath, shortness of	Iron
Breast-feeding	Calcium
Bronchitis, chronic	Sulphur
Bruises, frequent	Vitamin B_2
Burns	Vitamin E, potassium, silicon, copper
Cancer	Vitamin F, germanium, magnesium, selenium
Canned-food abuse	Selenium
Cellulitis	Iodine, silicon
Children	Calcium, iron

Cholesterol	Vitamins B5, B15, chromium, magnesium, zinc
Cicatrization, slow	Silicon, sulphur
Circulation	Vitamin B1, germanium
Cirrhosis	Zinc
Urban environment	Iron, selenium, magnesium
Coffee	Calcium, potassium
Colitis	Iron, potassium
Complexion, pallid	Cobalt
Concentration	Iron, manganese, phosphorus, zinc
Conjunctivitis	Vitamin B6
Constipation	Vitamin B7, choline, iron, fluoride, potassium, magnesium
Oral contraceptives	Calcium, iron, zinc, copper
Contusions	Vitamin F
Convalescence	Phosphorus
Cystitis	Vitamins A, D, E
Dandruff	Selenium
Decalcification	Phosphorus
Demineralization	Iodine, calcium, fluoride, molybdenum, phosphorus, silicon

Dental cavities	Calcium, fluoride, magnesium, molybdenum, phosphorus
Dentures	Calcium
Depression	Vitamins B_1, B_6, B_{12}, B_{17}, magnesium, zinc, calcium
Dermatosis	Vitamins B_2, B_3, sulphur
Diabetes	Vitamins A, E, chromium, manganese, potassium, zinc, selenium, magnesium
Diarrhea	Vitamins B_2, B_5, B_{12}, F, cobalt, potassium
Digestive problems	Vitamins B_1, B_2, copper, potassium
Eczema	Vitamins A, B_5, B_7, D, F, iodine, sulphur, calcium, copper
Elocution, difficult	Vitamin B_{12}
Epilepsy	Manganese
Eyes	Vitamin B_1, molybdenum, zinc
Fatigue	Vitamins B_3, B_5, B_6, B_{12}, B_{15}, cobalt, iron, manganese, phosphorus, potassium, zinc, magnesium
Fertility	Vitamin F, selenium
Fever	Sodium
Frozen food	Selenium

Gall bladder	Sulphur
Gall stones	Vitamins F, H
Gingivitis	Phosphorus
Goitre	Iodine
Gout	Vitamin F
Growth	Vitamin B_2, calcium, phosphorus, copper, fluoride, magnesium, potassium, silicon
Hair, brittle	Silicon
Hair, dry	Iodine
Hair, gray	Vitamin B_{10}, F, calcium
Hair loss	Vitamins B_5, B_6, B_7, E, F, iron
Headaches	Vitamins A, E
Heart	Vitamins A, F
Heart attack	Chromium, copper, germanium, magnesium, potassium, selenium
Hematomas	Vitamin H
Hemorrhages	Vitamin H, iron
Hemorrhoids	Iron
Hepatitis	Vitamin A

Hypertension	Cobalt, magnesium, potassium, calcium, selenium, chromium, germanium
Hypoglycemia	Vitamin B5, chromium, manganese
Hypotension	Vitamin B5
Immunity	Copper, manganese, selenium, zinc, magnesium, sulphur
Infections	Vitamins B5, F
Influenza	Germanium, magnesium
Insomnia	Vitamin B3, calcium, magnesium, potassium
Intestinal pains	Vitamin B3, B9
Insect bites	Magnesium
Kidneys	Phosphorus, silicon
Kidney stones	Magnesium
Laryngitis	Sulphur
Liver troubles	Choline, sulphur
Medications	Vitamin F
Memory	Vitamin B3, B6, choline
Men	Zinc, selenium
Menopause	Vitamin E, calcium

Menstrual cramps	Vitamins B6, E, F, H, calcium, calcium, iron, magnesium
Mental problems	Vitamin B1
Migraines	Vitamin E, magnesium, molybdenum, calcium, silicon
Mood disorders	Vitamin B12
Multiple sclerosis	Vitamin F, germanium
Muscles	Manganese, selenium
Muscle pains	Vitamins B3, B5
Muscular cramps	Calcium, sodium, potassium, magnesium
Myopathy	Germanium
Myopia	Vitamin E
Nails, brittle	Calcium, iron, silicon, zinc
Nausea	Molybdenum
Nettle rash	Sulphur
Nervous system	Copper, phosphorus, sodium, calcium, cobalt, magnesium
Nervousness	Vitamins B1, B3, B6, B12, F, calcium, fluoride, iodine, magnesium, manganese, potassium
Numbness of limbs	Calcium, iodine

Obesity	Vitamin E, calcium, fluoride, iodine, magnesium, phosphorus, chromium, silicon
Palpitations	Calcium, cobalt
Parkinson's disease	Germanium
Sore throat	Sulphur
Phlebitis	Vitamin E
Photophobia	Vitamin B$_2$
Pollution	Vitamin F
Pregnancy	Magnesium, calcium
Prostate	Magnesium, zinc
Psoriasis	Vitamins A, D, F, sulphur, calcium, zinc, selenium, magnesium
Rickets	Calcium, fluoride, phosphorus, magnesium, silicon
Rheumatism	Vitamin E, F, calcium, germanium, iodine, zinc, selenium, magnesium, copper, manganese
Ringing in the ears	Manganese
Scars	Vitamin E
Scoliosis	Fluoride
Sinusitis	Vitamins A, E
Skin, dry	Vitamin F, B$_9$, iron, potassium, zinc

Skin diseases	Copper, sulphur, silicon
Spasmophillia	Phosphorus, calcium, cobalt
Sports	Vitamins A, B15, magnesium, potassium
Sterility, men	Zinc
Stomach pains	Vitamins B3, B5, B9
Stomach ulcers	Choline
Stress	Vitamins A, D, E, calcium, iodine, magnesium, phosphorus
Sun sensitivity	Vitamin B3
Teeth	Vitamin A
Thirst, exaggerated	Vitamin F
Throat inflammation	Sodium
Thrombosis	Vitamins E, F
Ulcers	Iron, zinc, germanium
Uric acid	Phosphorus
Varicose veins	Vitamins E, F, copper, magnesium, calcium
Vegetarians	Zinc
Vertigo	Vitamin B2, manganese
Vomiting	Vitamin B5, molybdenum, sodium
Warts	Vitamin E

Women	Iron
Wounds	Silicon, zinc
Wrinkles	Vitamins B_{10}, E, zinc, silicon